A FRANCESCA

ATLAS OF

UROLOGIC SURGERY

VOLUME I

ORTHOTOPIC

URINARY DIVERSION

FABRIZIO DAL MORO

UNIVERSITY OF PADOVA

ASSISTANT PROFESSOR

UROLOGY

PADOVA

FABRIZIO DAL MORO
UNIVERSITY OF PADOVA
VIA GIUSTINIANI 2
35126 – PADOVA
E-MAIL: *FABRIZIO.DALMORO@UNIPD.IT*

2015 EDITION

ISBN-13: 978-1517286118
ISBN-10: 1517286115

ATLAS OF

UROLOGIC SURGERY

VOLUME I

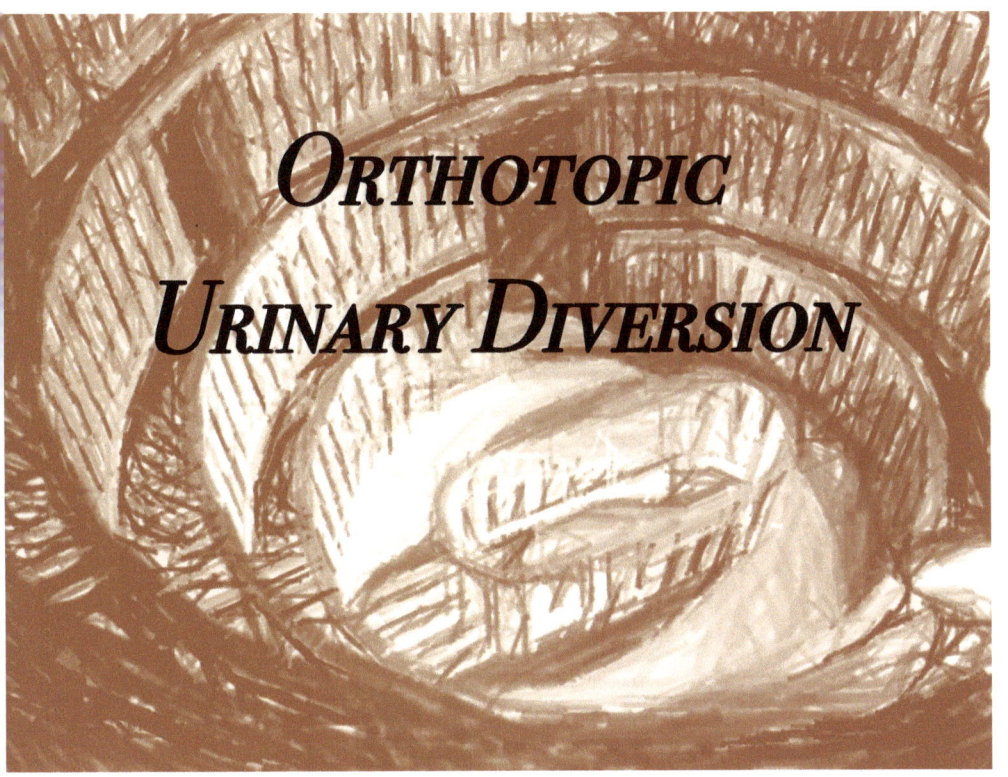

ORTHOTOPIC

URINARY DIVERSION

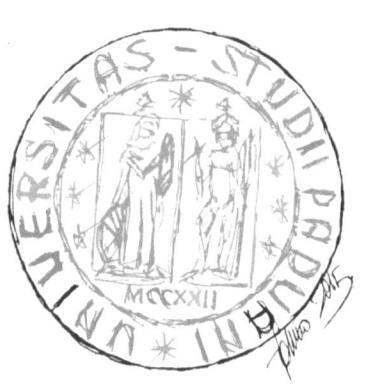

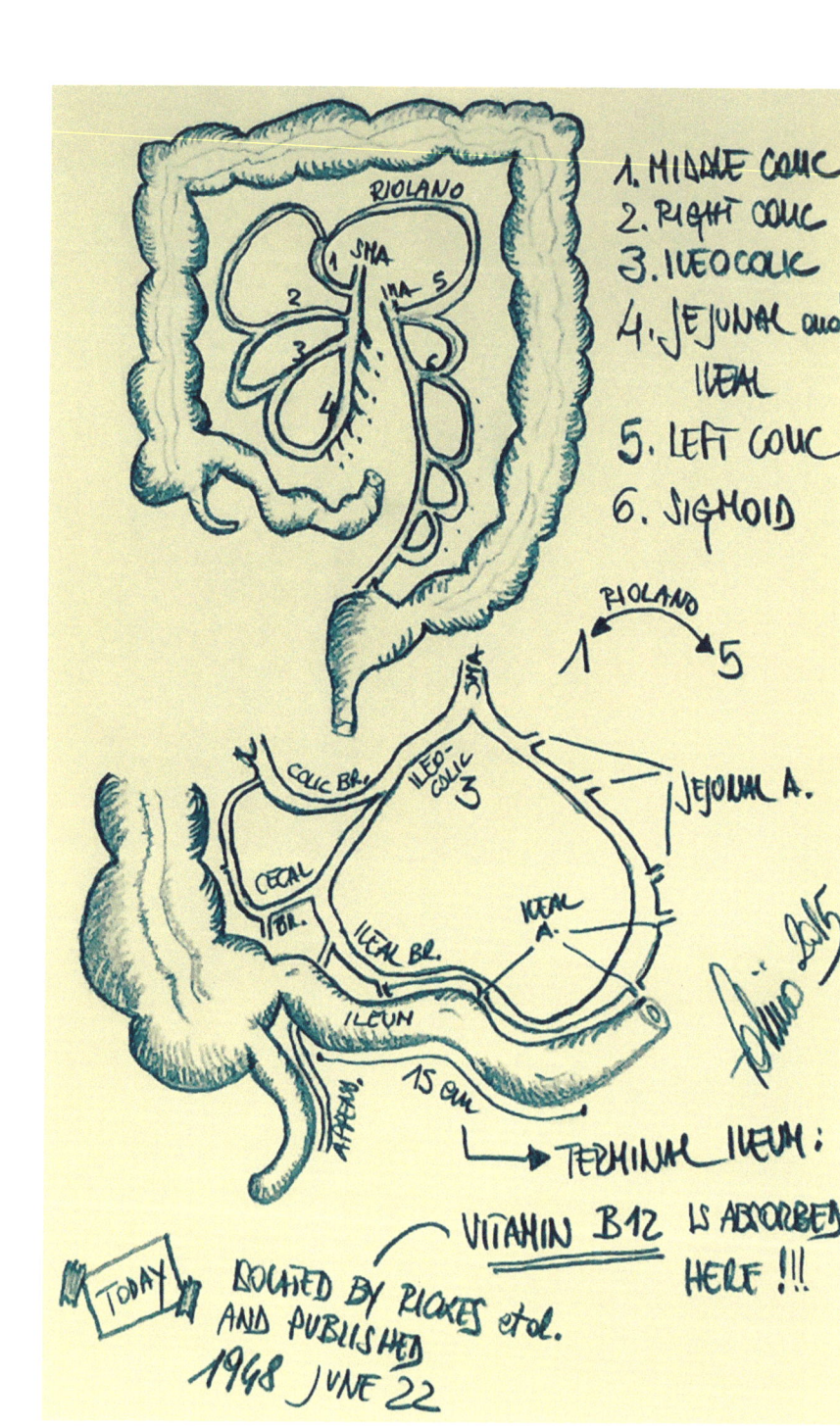

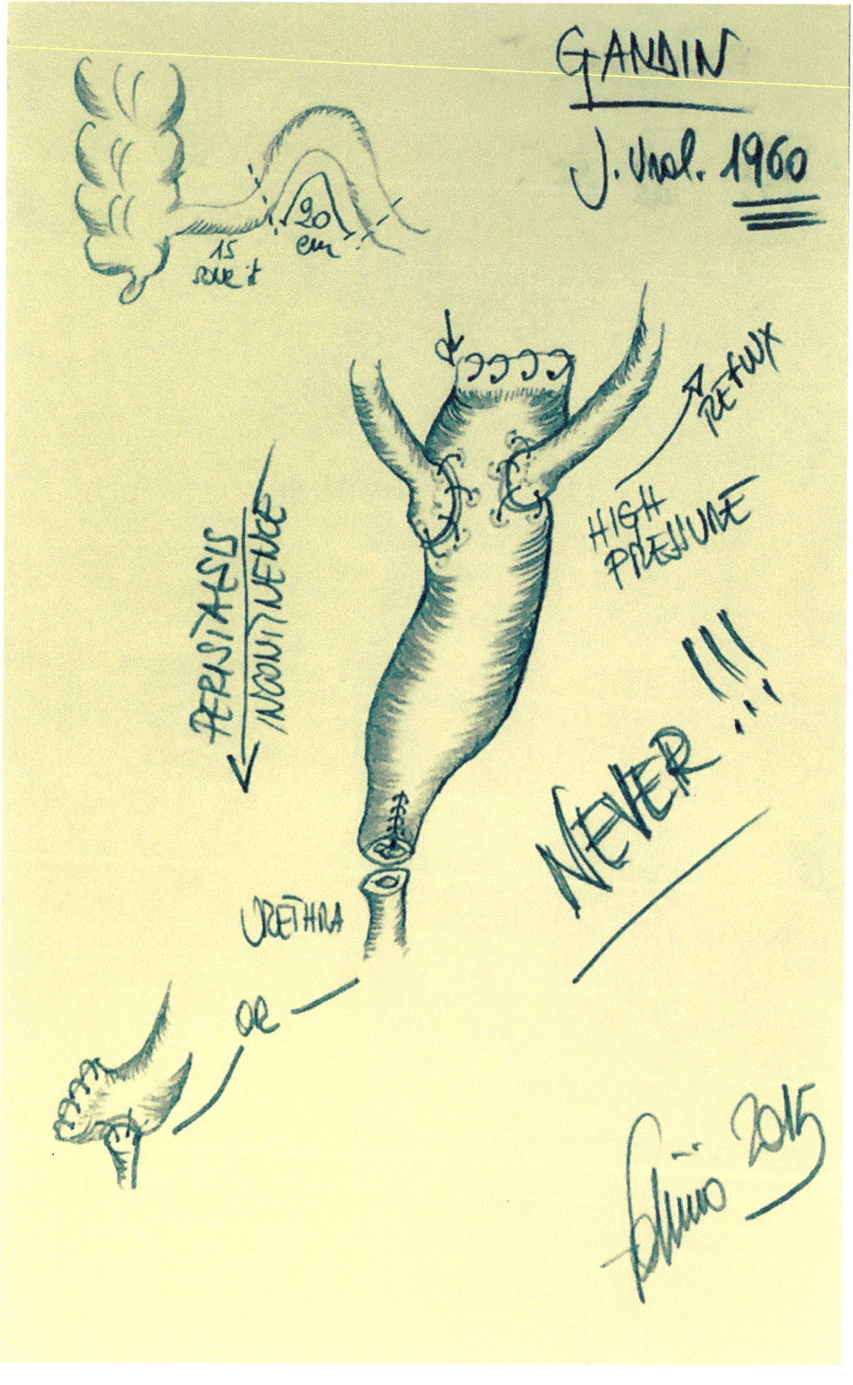

GANDIN
J. Urol. 1960
15
20 cm
REFLUX
HIGH PRESSURE
PERISTALSIS
INCONTINENCE
NEVER !!!
URETHRA
OR
2015

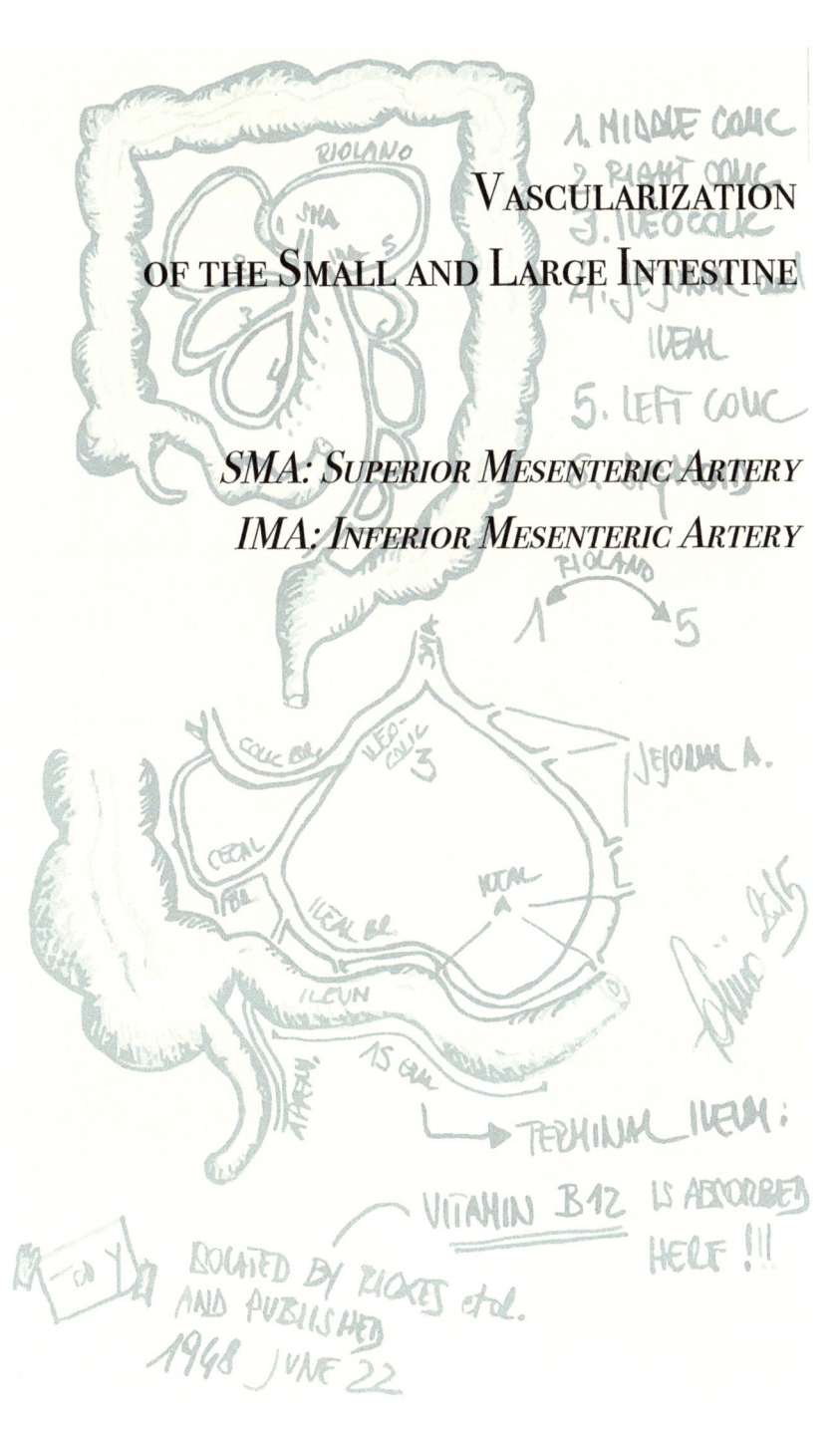

Vascularization
of the Small and Large Intestine

SMA: Superior Mesenteric Artery
IMA: Inferior Mesenteric Artery

Bladder Substitution
According to Gandin (1960)

CAMEY 1

Eur. Urol. 1979

440 cm

URETHRA

Folino 2015

Bladder Substitution According to Camey and LeDuc (1979)

CAMEY I

EUR. URO. 1979

40 cm

URETHRA

Silvio 2015

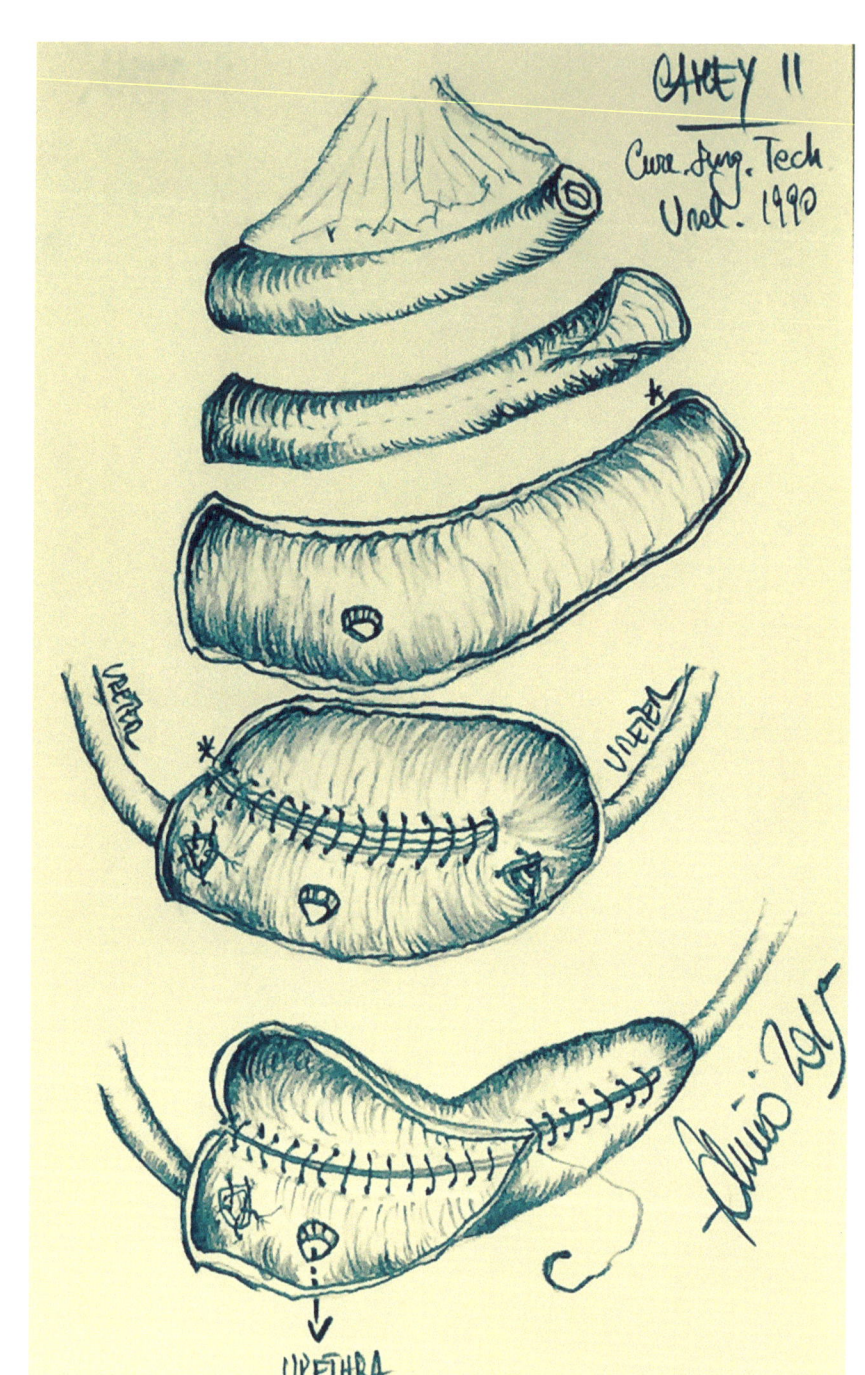

BLADDER SUBSTITUTION ACCORDING TO CAMEY (1990)

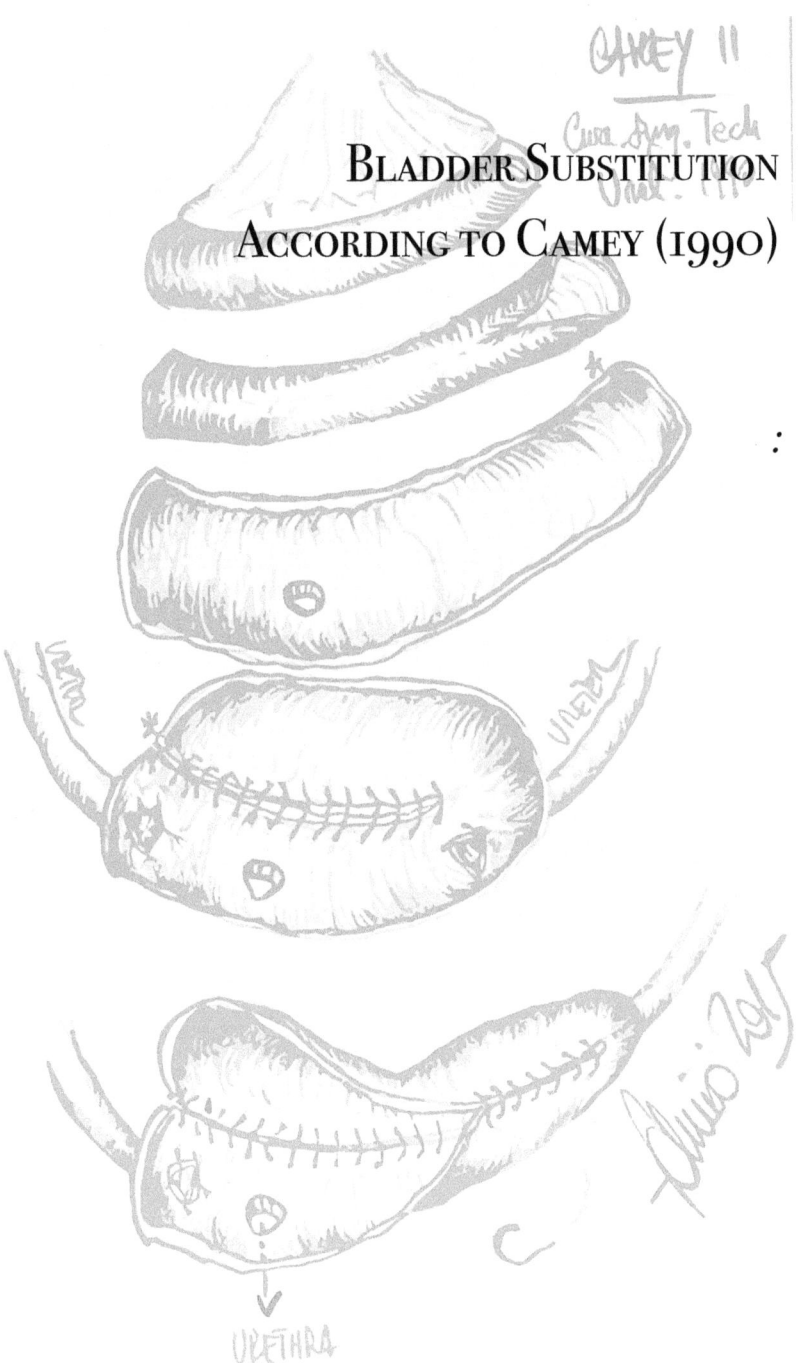

MAINZ
J. Urol. 1986

RIGHT URETER
LEFT URETER

M . MIXED
A . AUGMENTATION
I . ILEUM
N . "N"
Z . ZECUM

URETHRAL
ANASTOMOSIS

Bladder Substitution
MAINZ (1986)

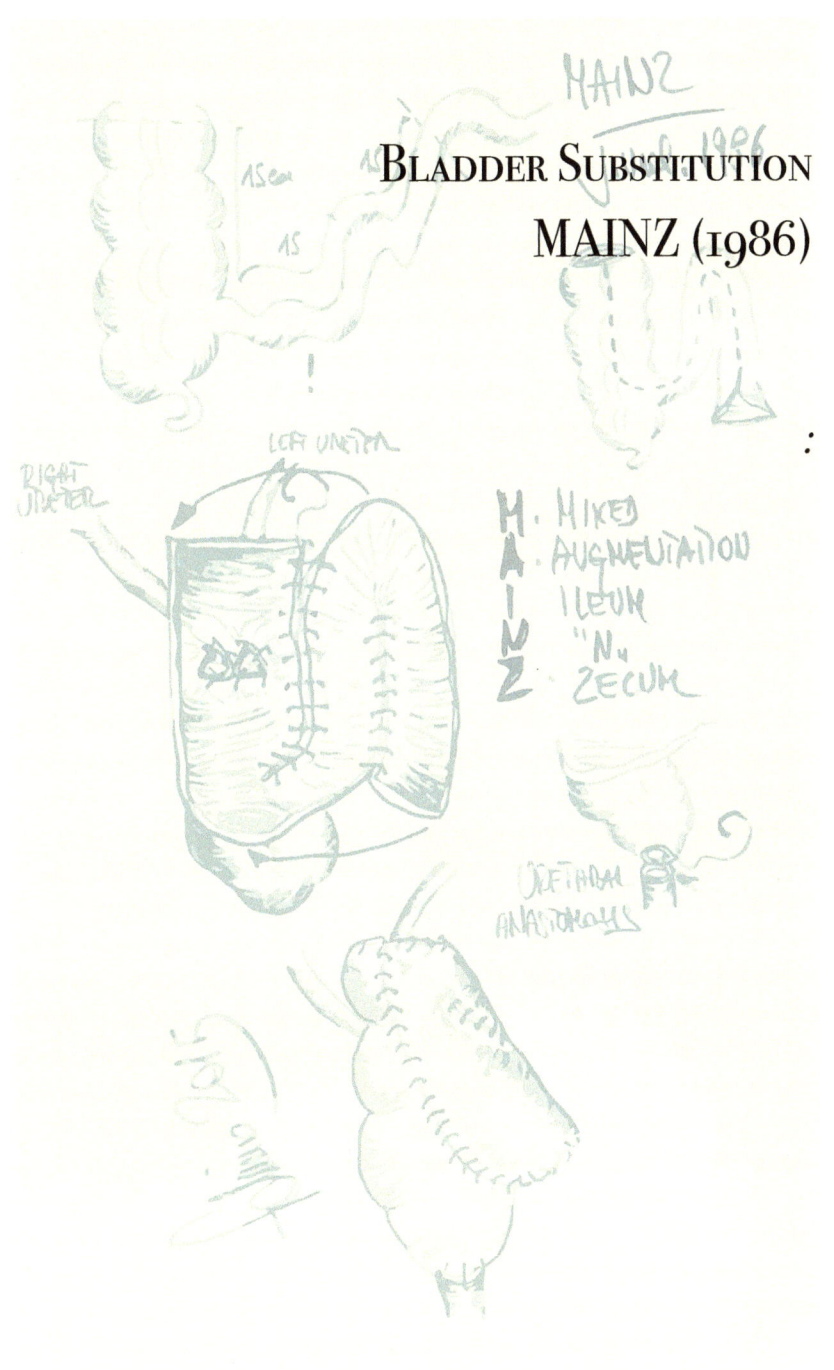

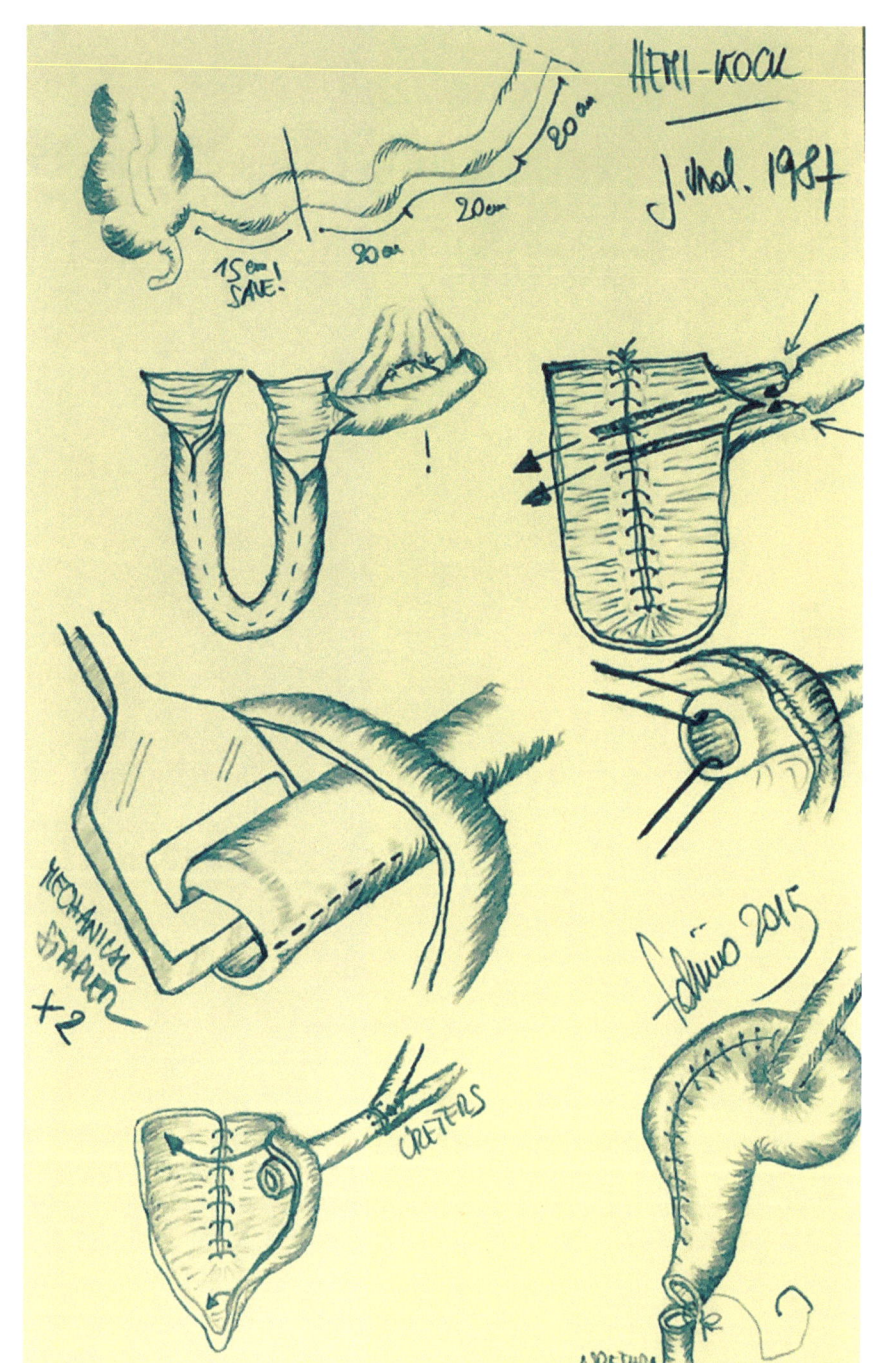

Bladder Substitution
Hemi-Kock (1987)

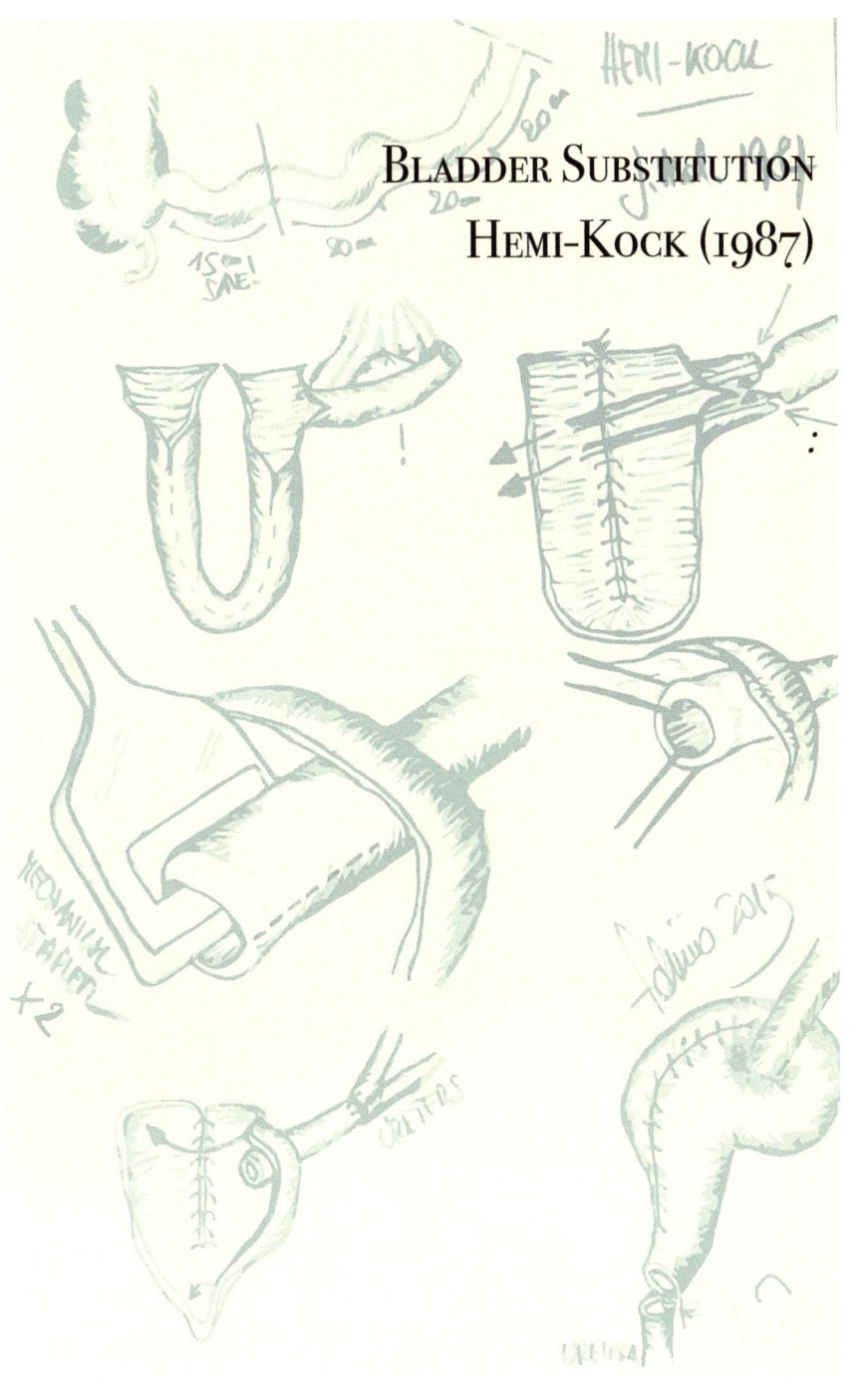

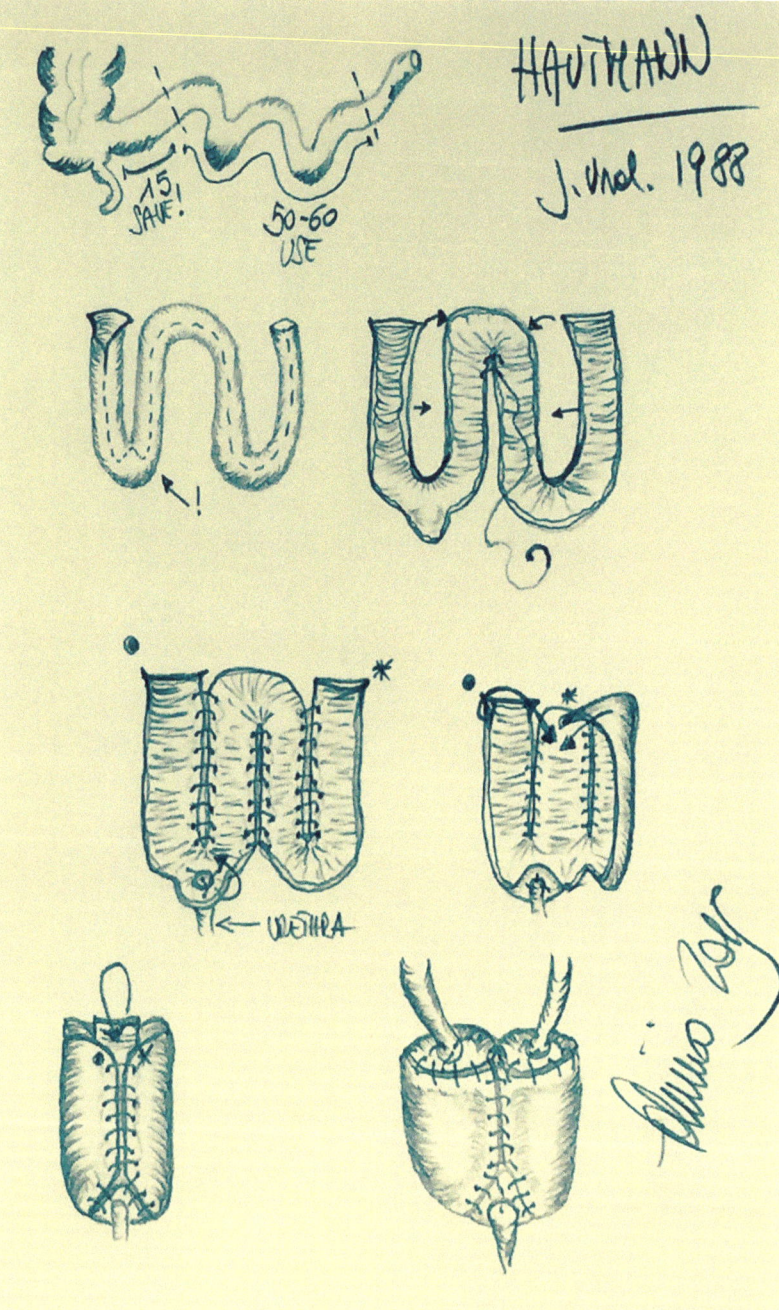

HAUTMANN

J. Urol. 1988

15 SAVE!

50-60 USE

← URETHRA

Bladder Substitution According to Hautmann (1988)

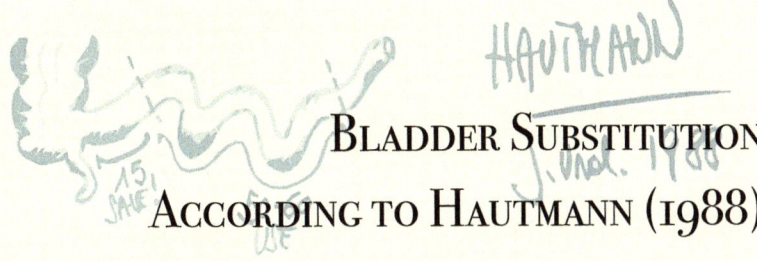

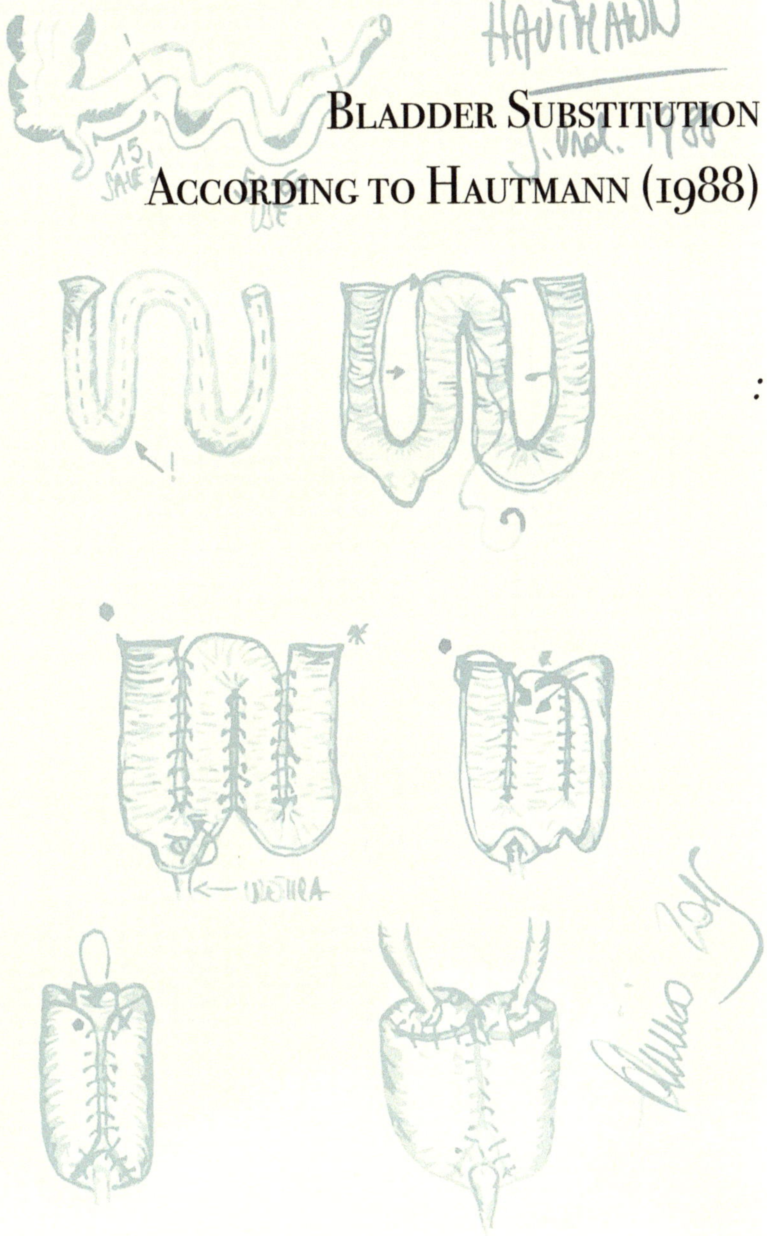

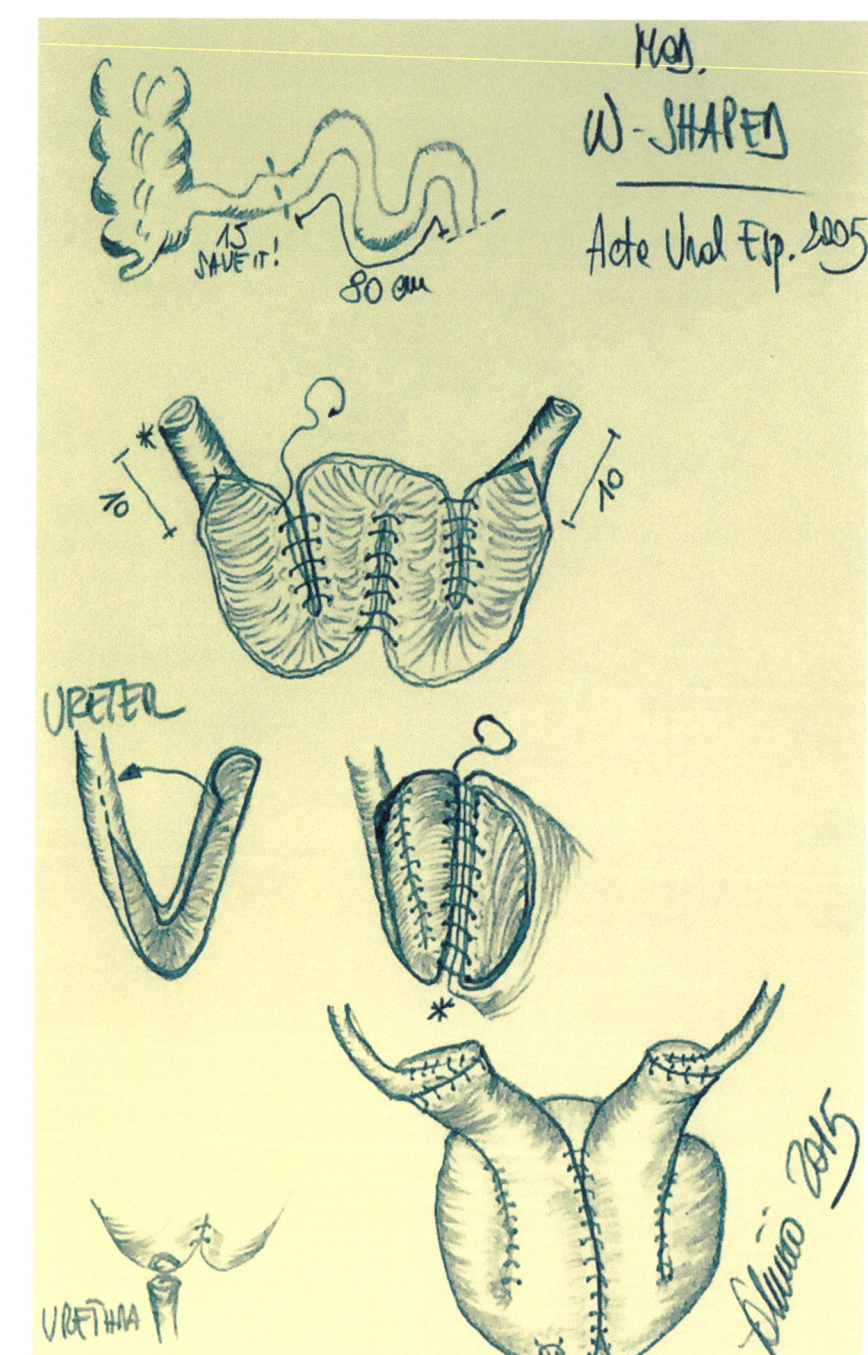

W-Shaped (Mod. 2005)

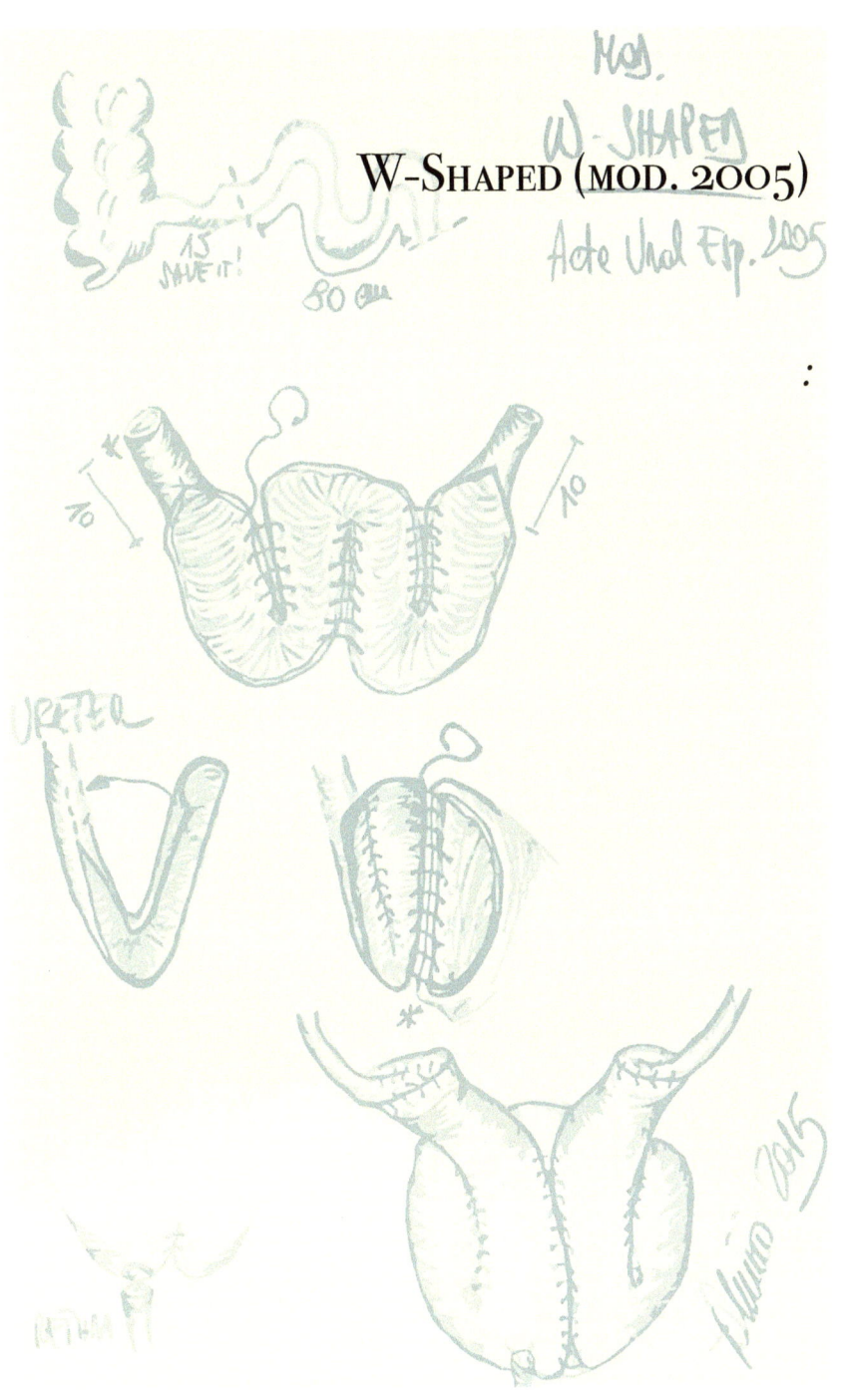

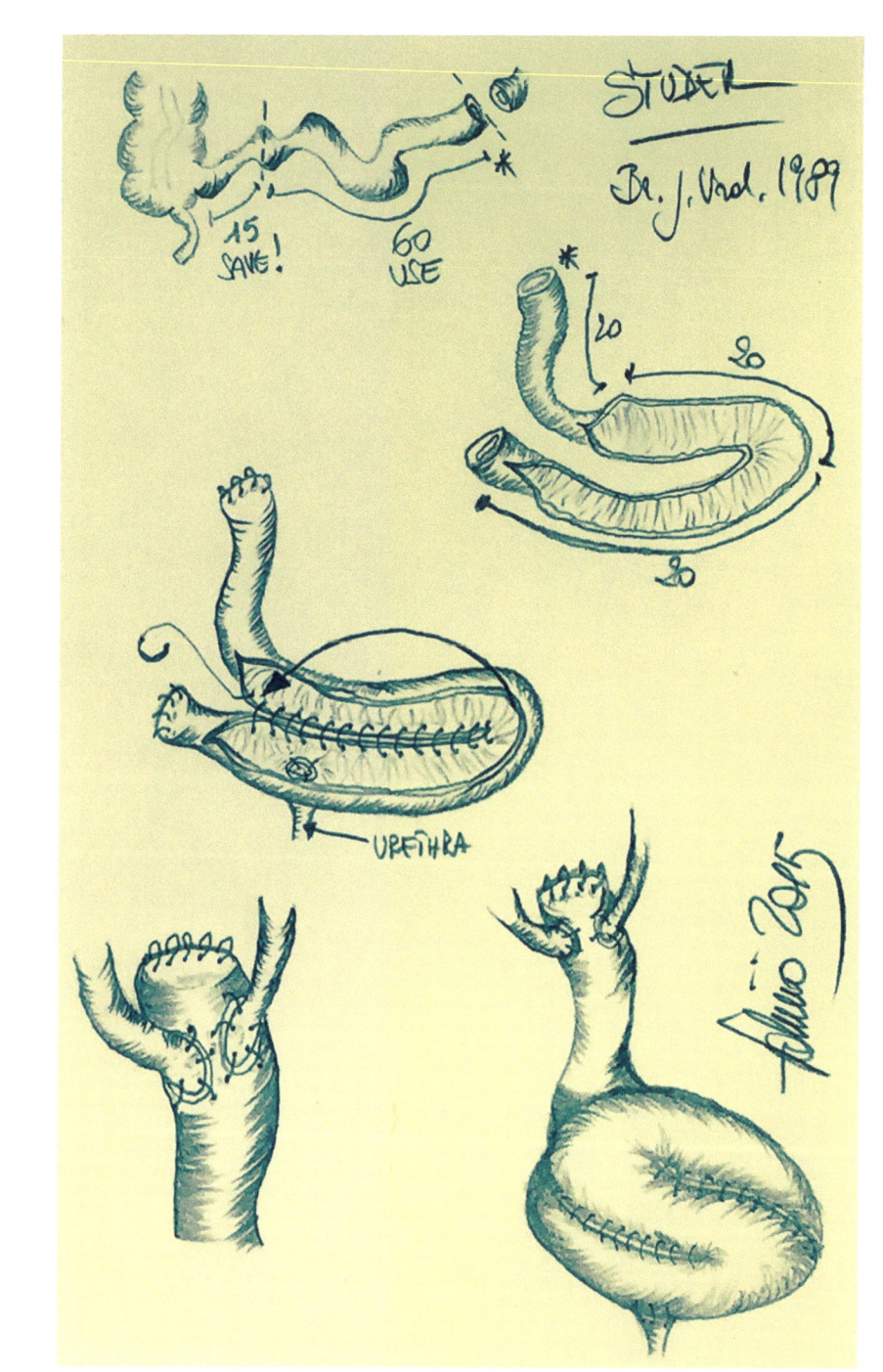

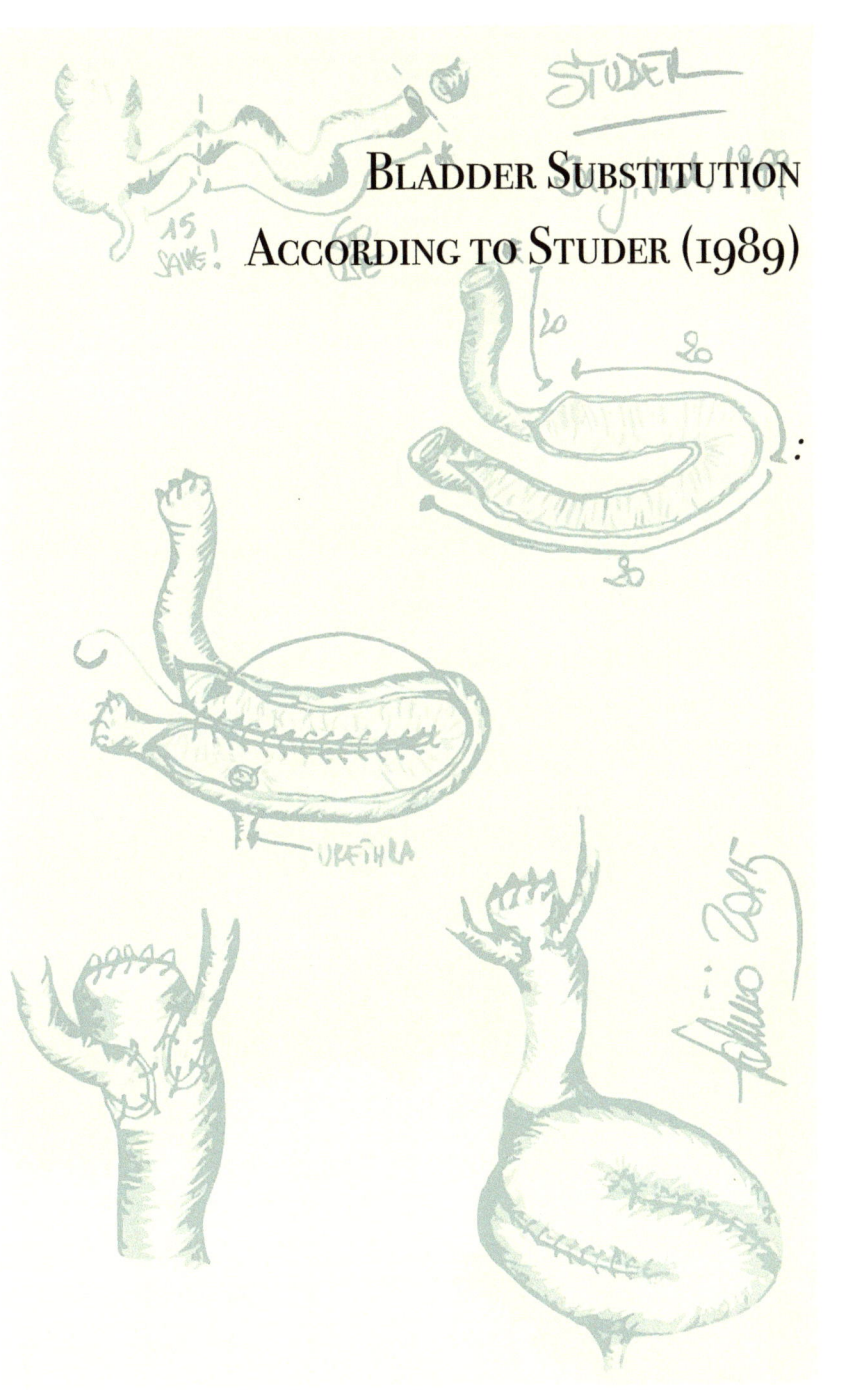

BLADDER SUBSTITUTION ACCORDING TO STUDER (1989)

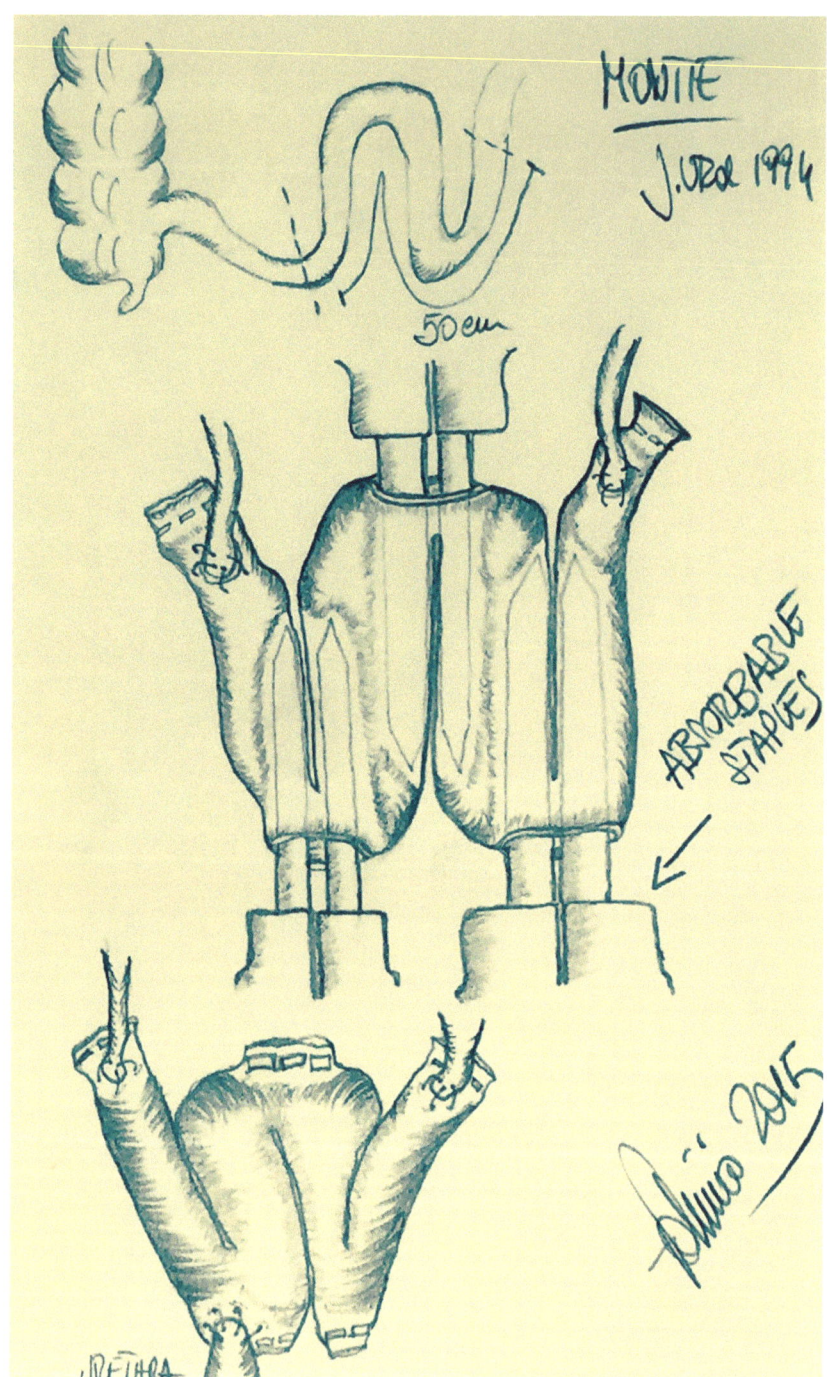

Bladder Substitution According to Montie (1994)

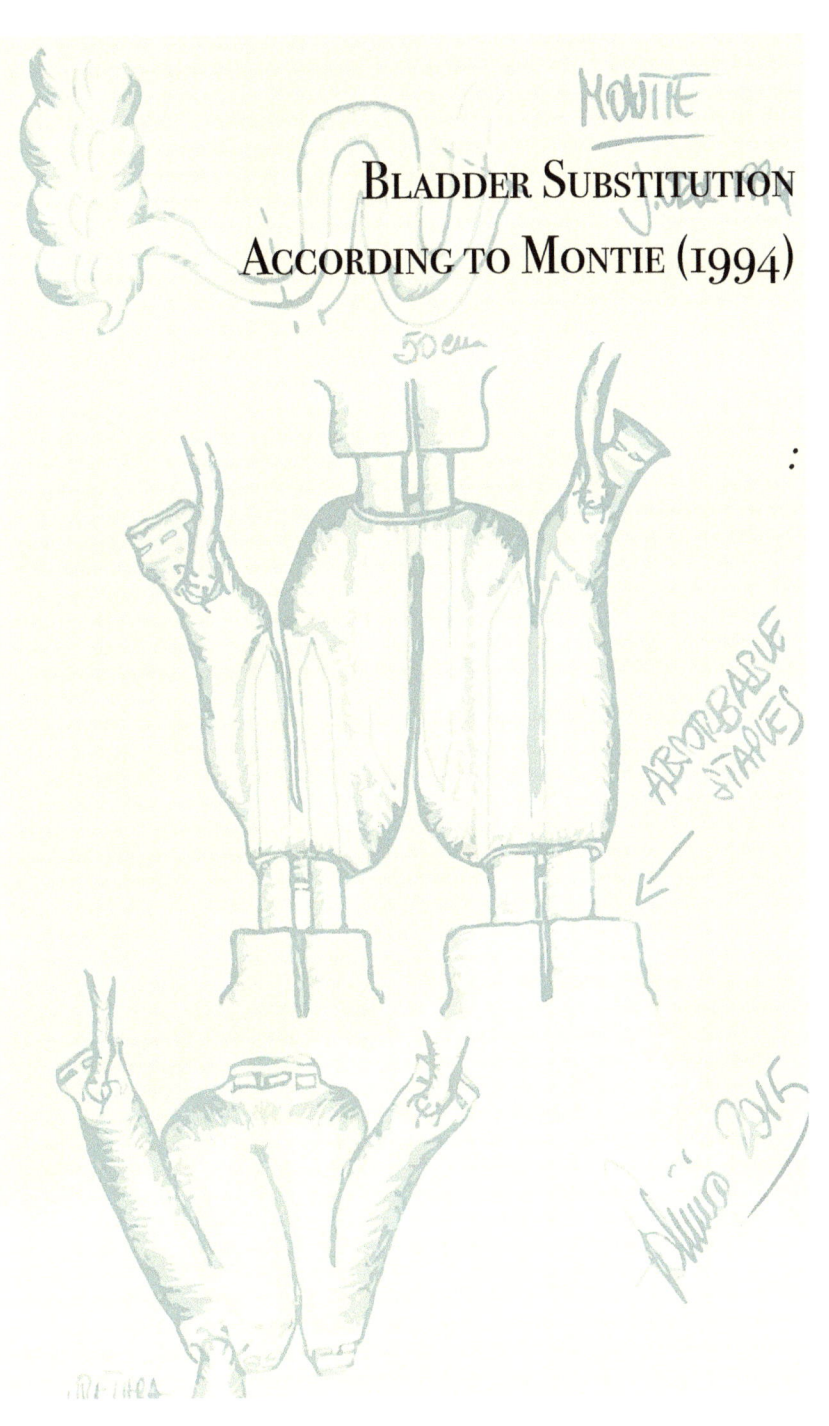

MODIFIED
U-SHAPED

Urol.Oncol 2013

15 cm

40 cm

URETHRA

Alim 2015

U-Shaped (mod. 2013)

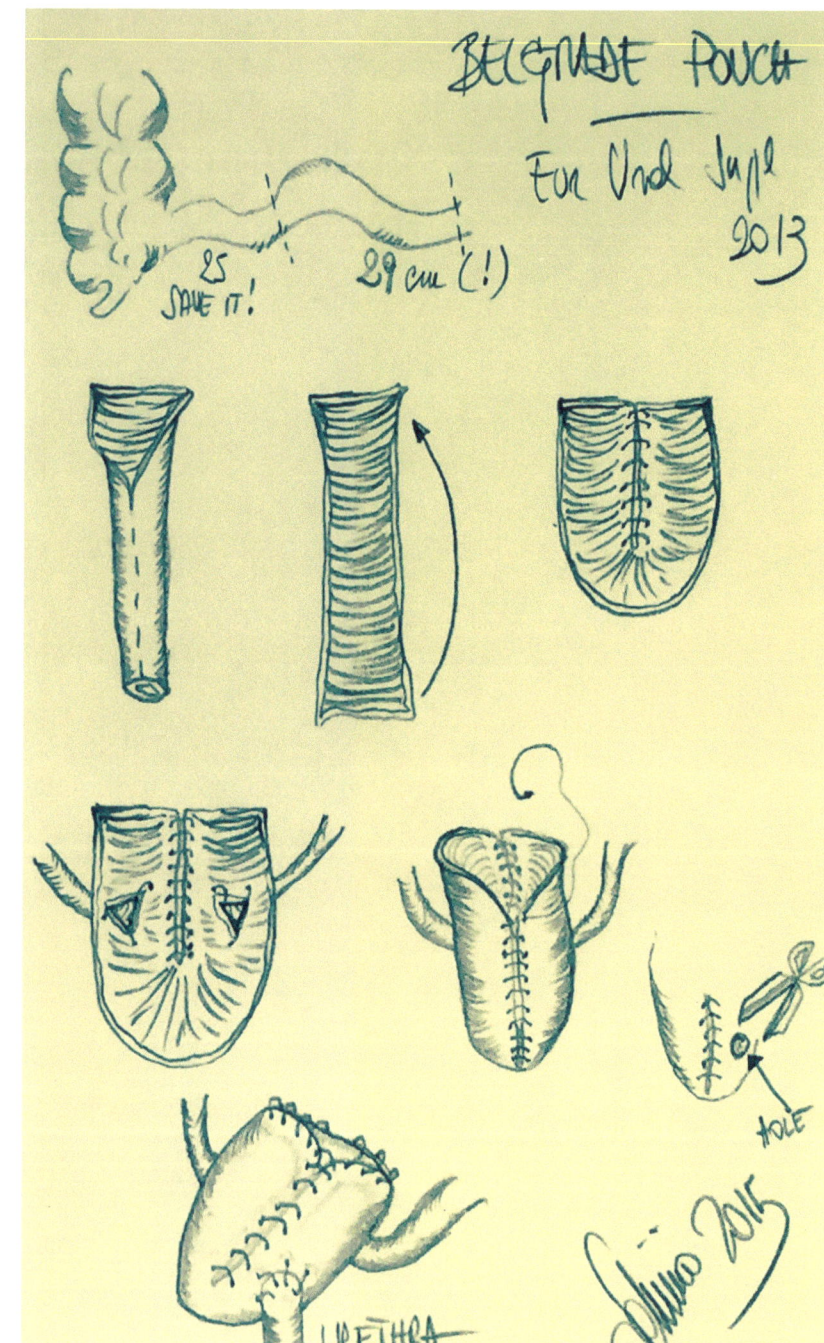

BELGRADE POUCH (2013)

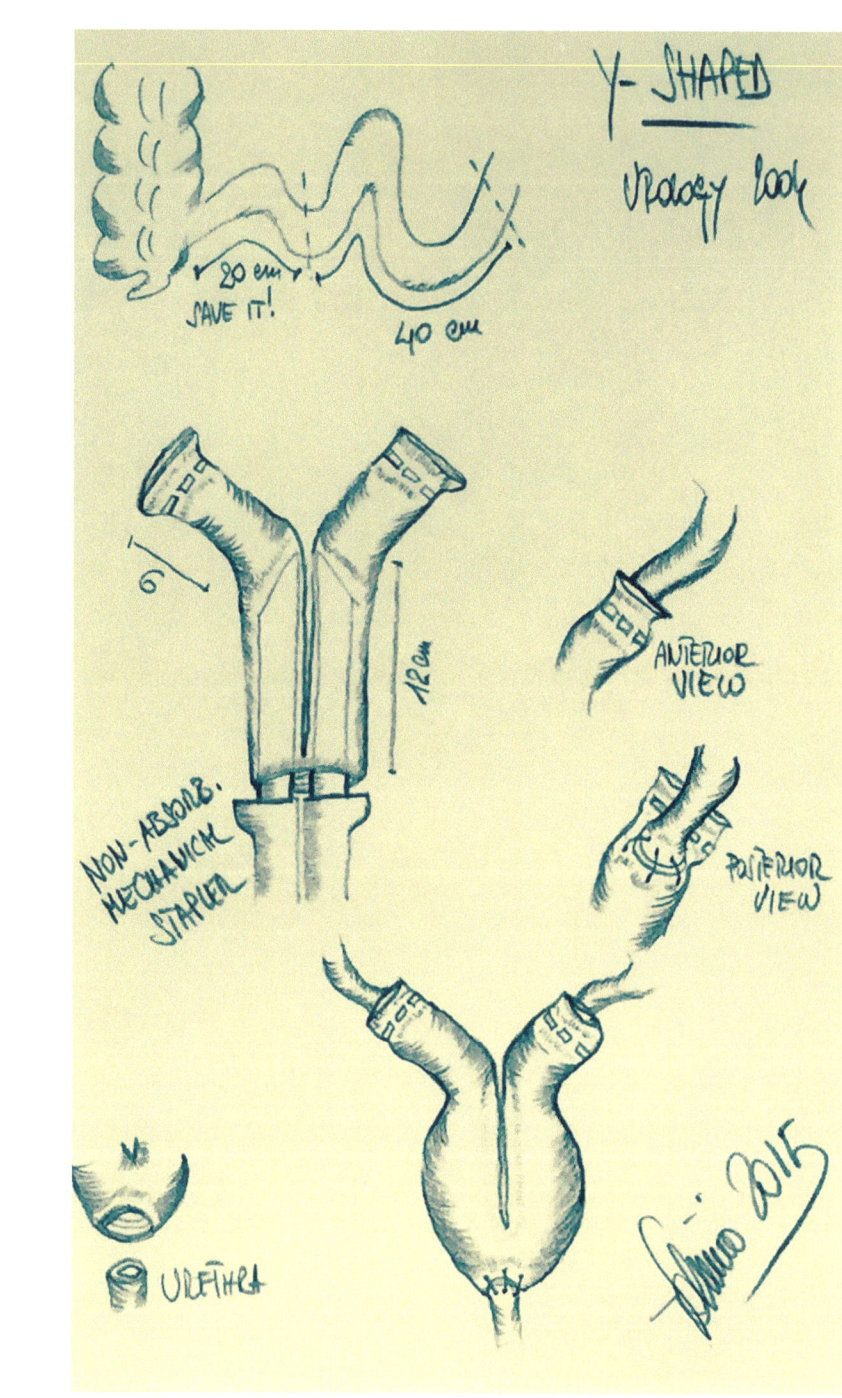

Y-Shaped (2004)

:

Y-ILEAL
NEOBLADDER
(TANTA - POUCH)

luth. Jund 2007

20cm
JAVE IT!

40cm

6   6

URETHRA

Jelmino 2015

Y-Ileal Neobladder
TANTA Pouch (2007)

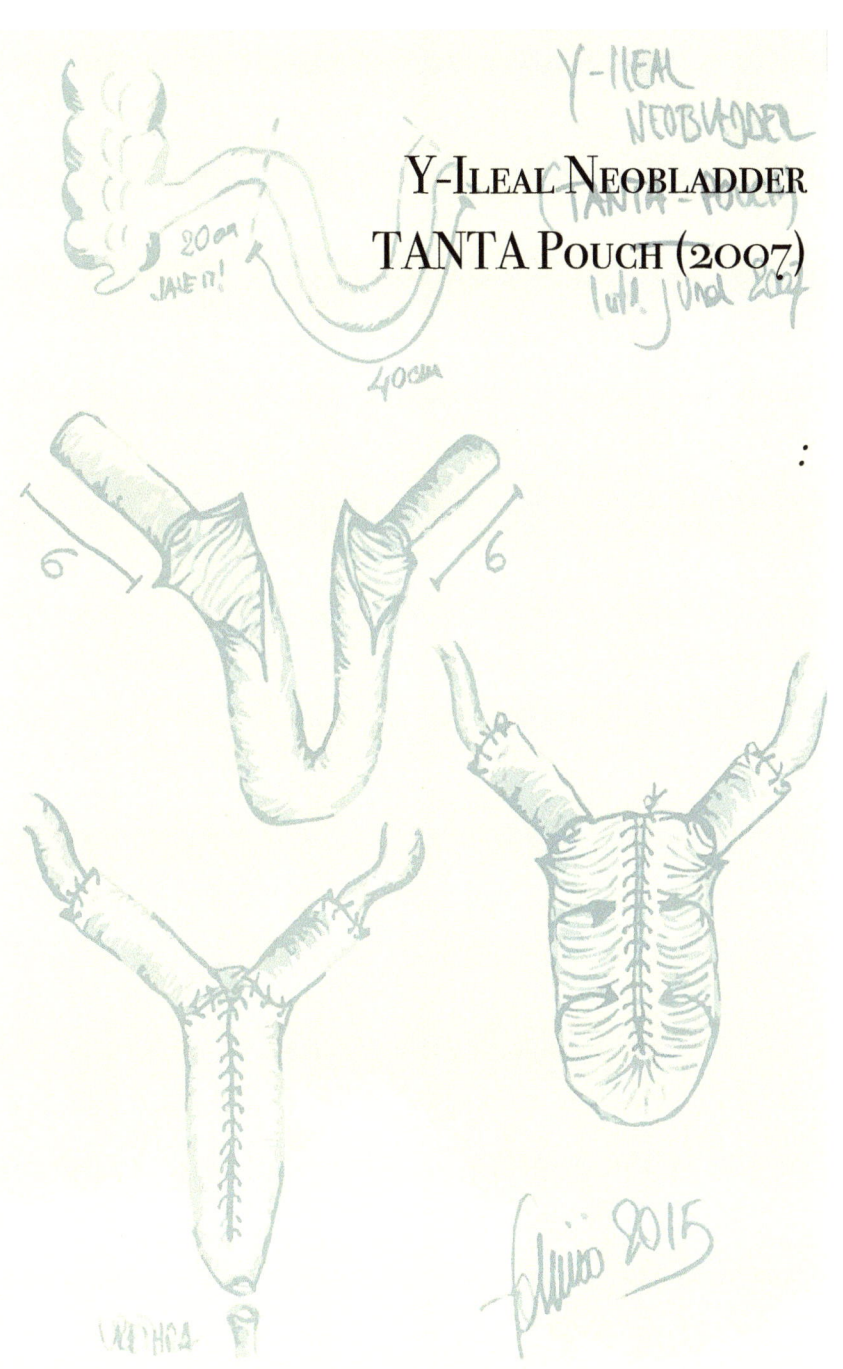

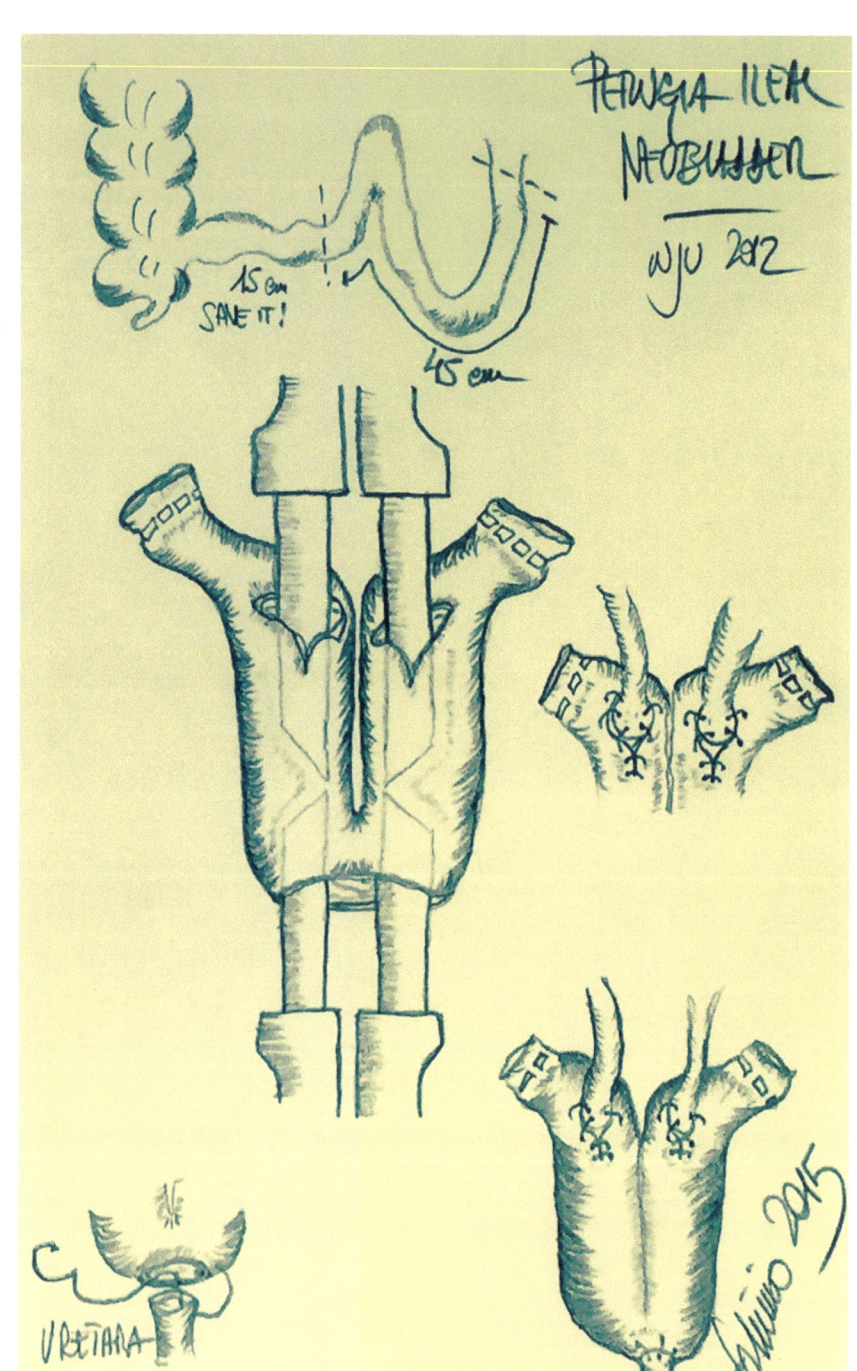

Perugia Ileal Neobladder (2012)

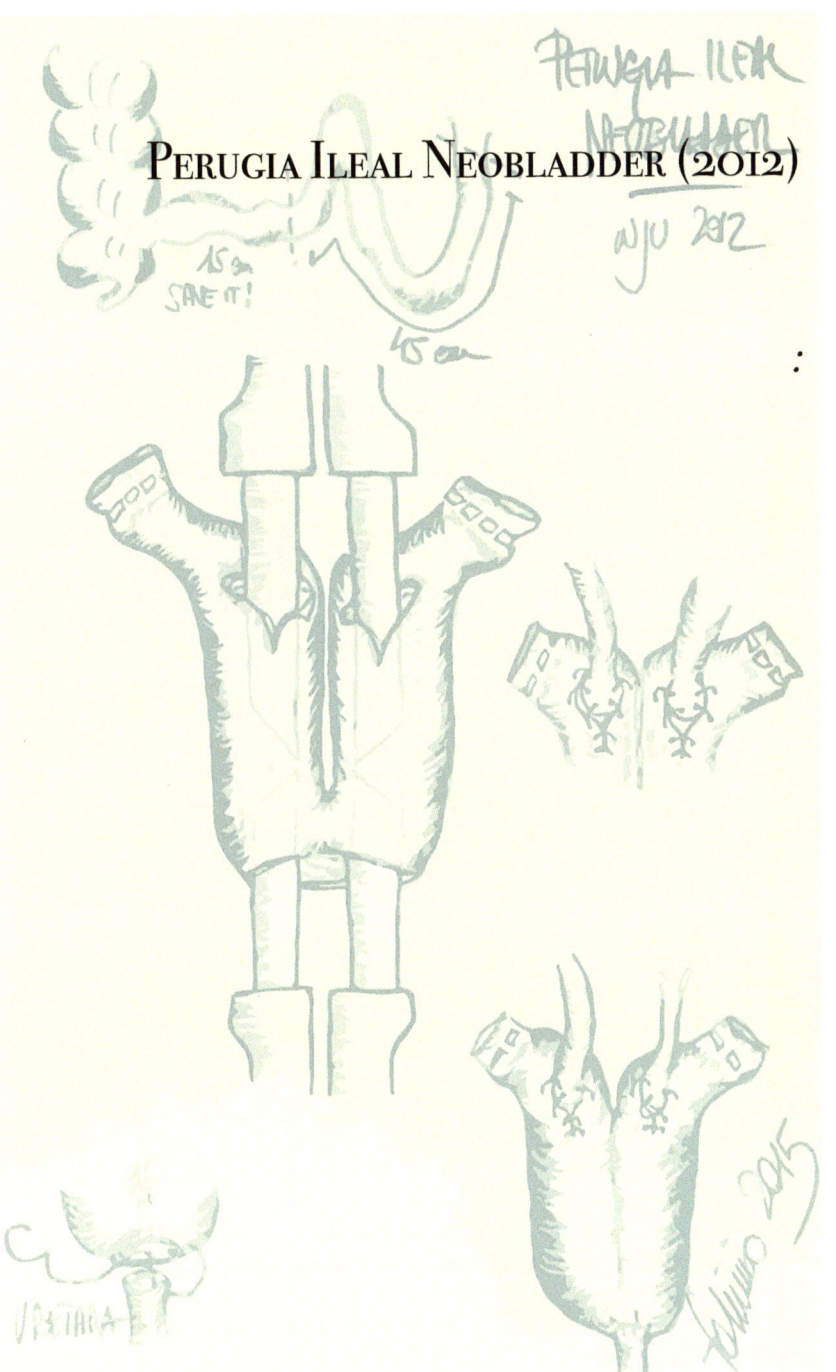

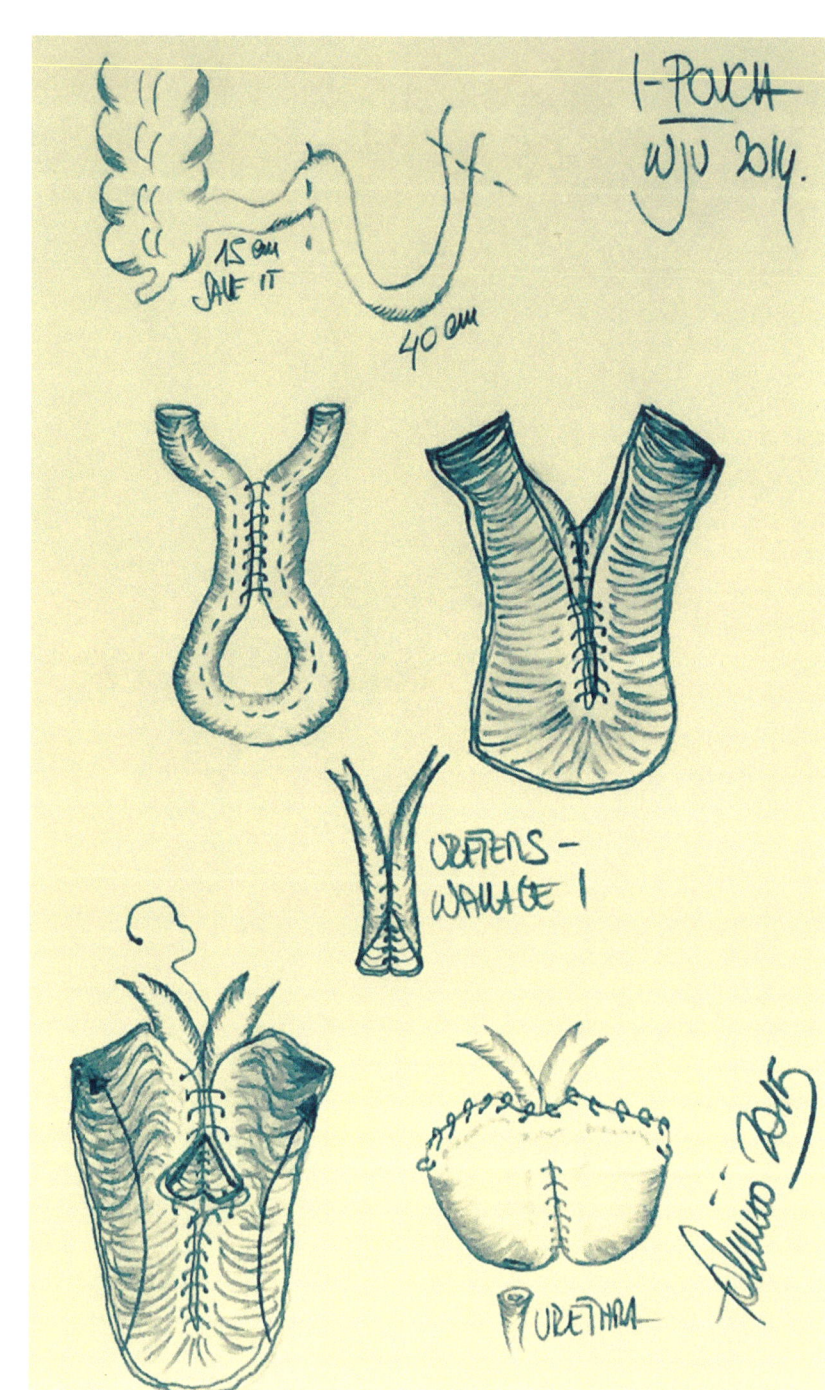

I-Pouch (2014)

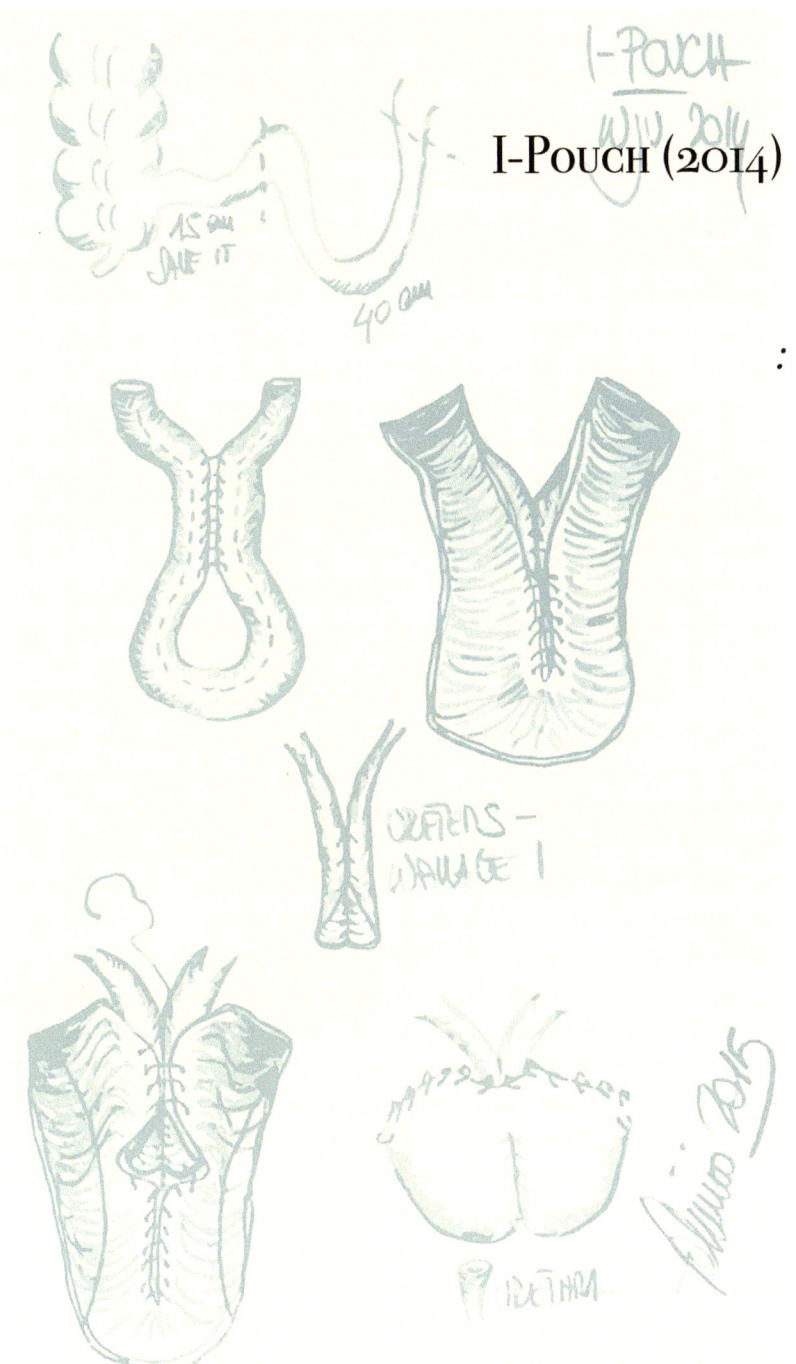

"PITCHER PLOT"

JPN J CLIN ONK.
2006

25 cm
SAVE IT

55 cm

15 cm

URETHRA

2015

PITCHER-PLOT (2006)

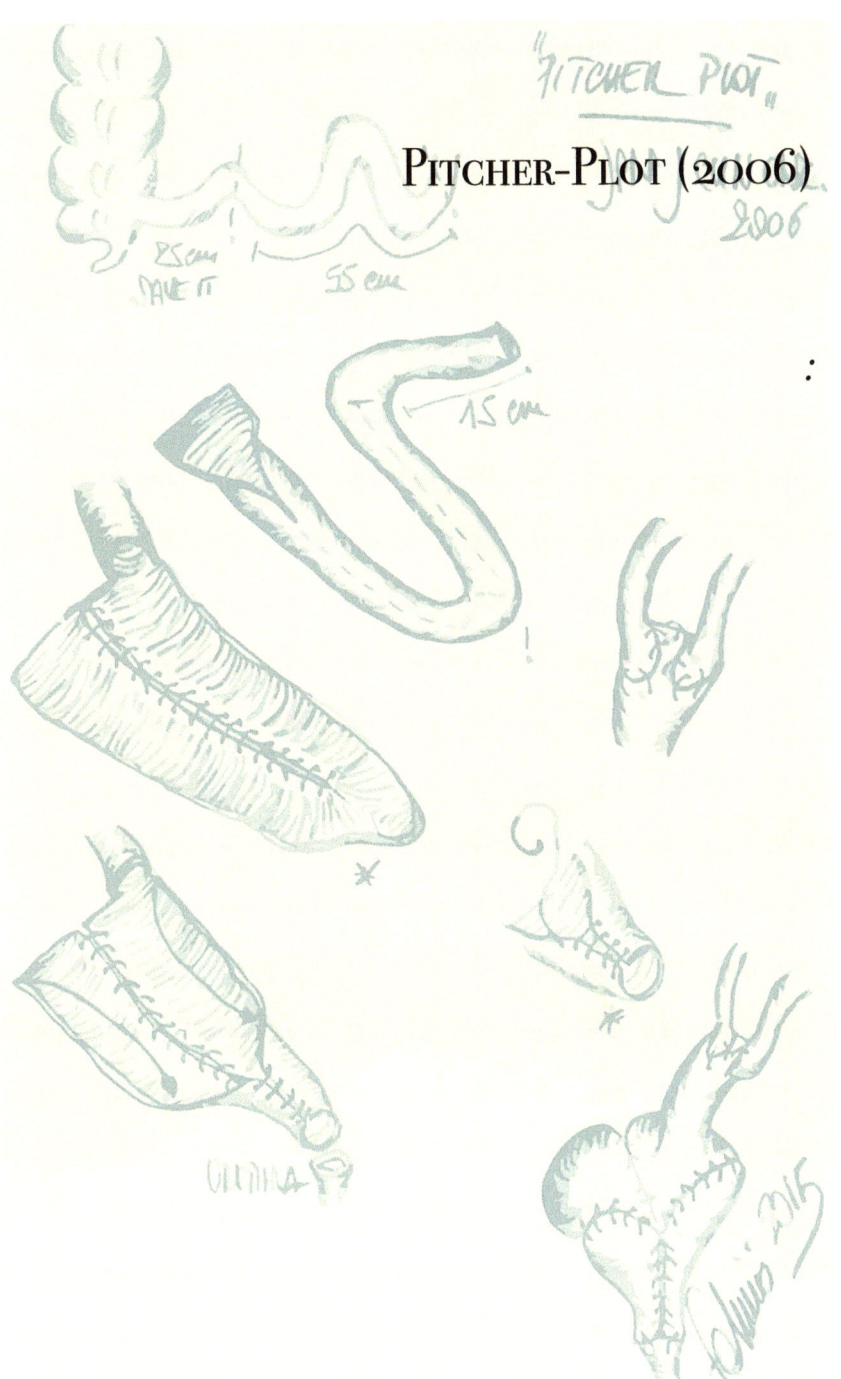

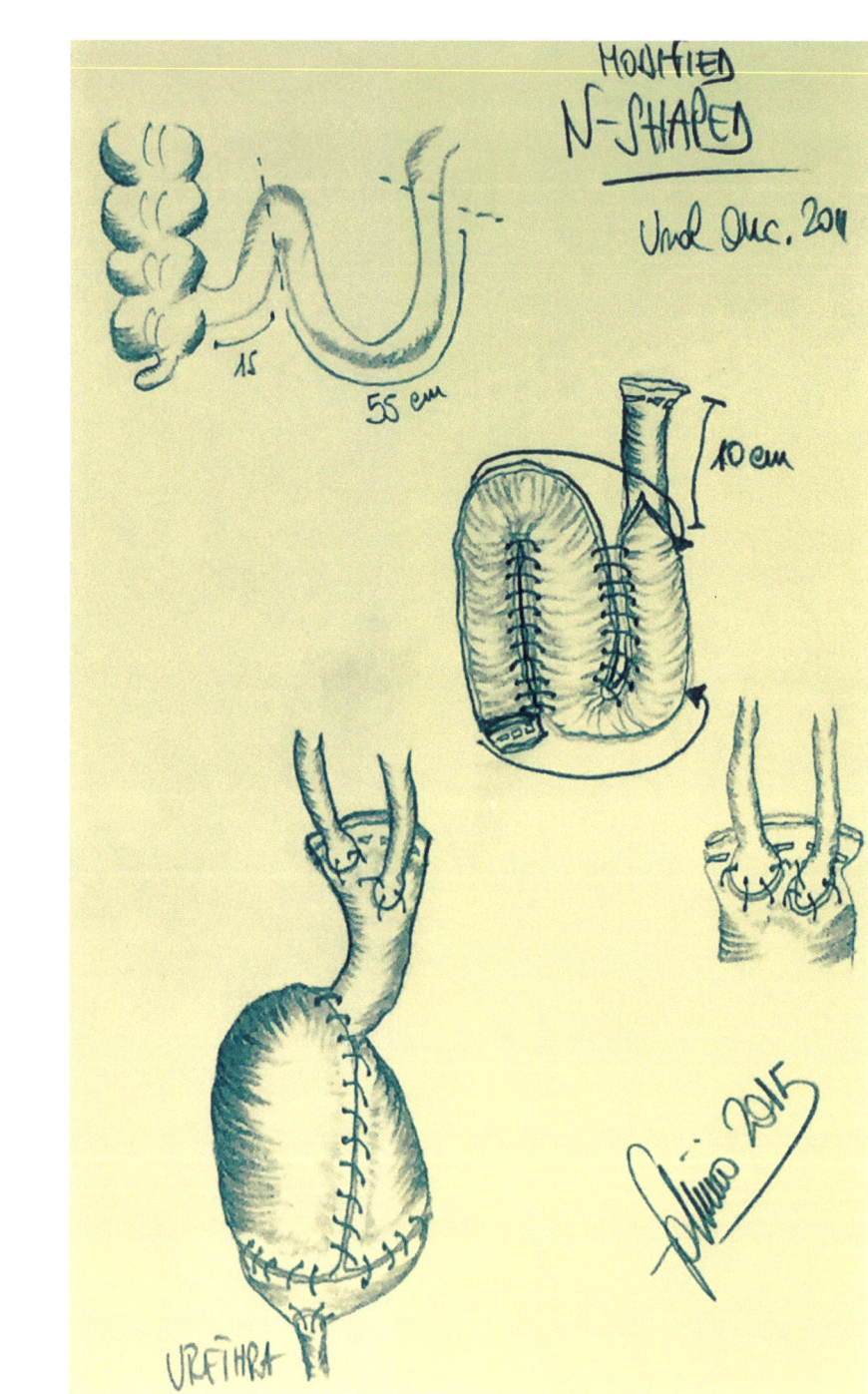

15

55 cm

10 cm

URETHRA

2015

N-Shaped (mod. 2011)

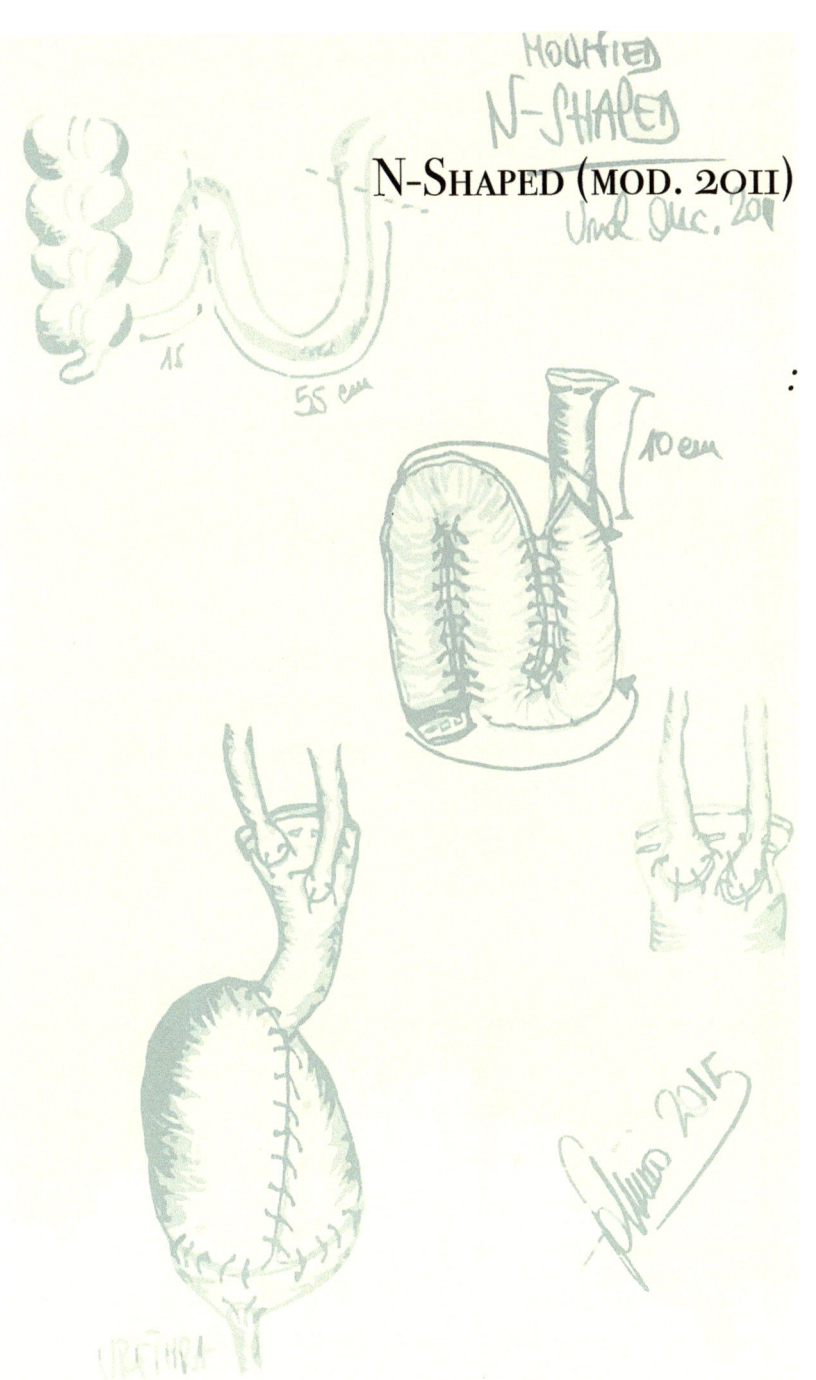

mod. S-SHAPED

EJSo 2008

30 cm
SAVE IT!

37 cm

6]
*

1]

URETHRA

2015

S-Shaped (mod. 2008)

Z-SHAPED
BJUI 2010

15.
SAVE IT!

45 cm

URETHRA

Silvio 2015

Z-Shaped (2010)

:

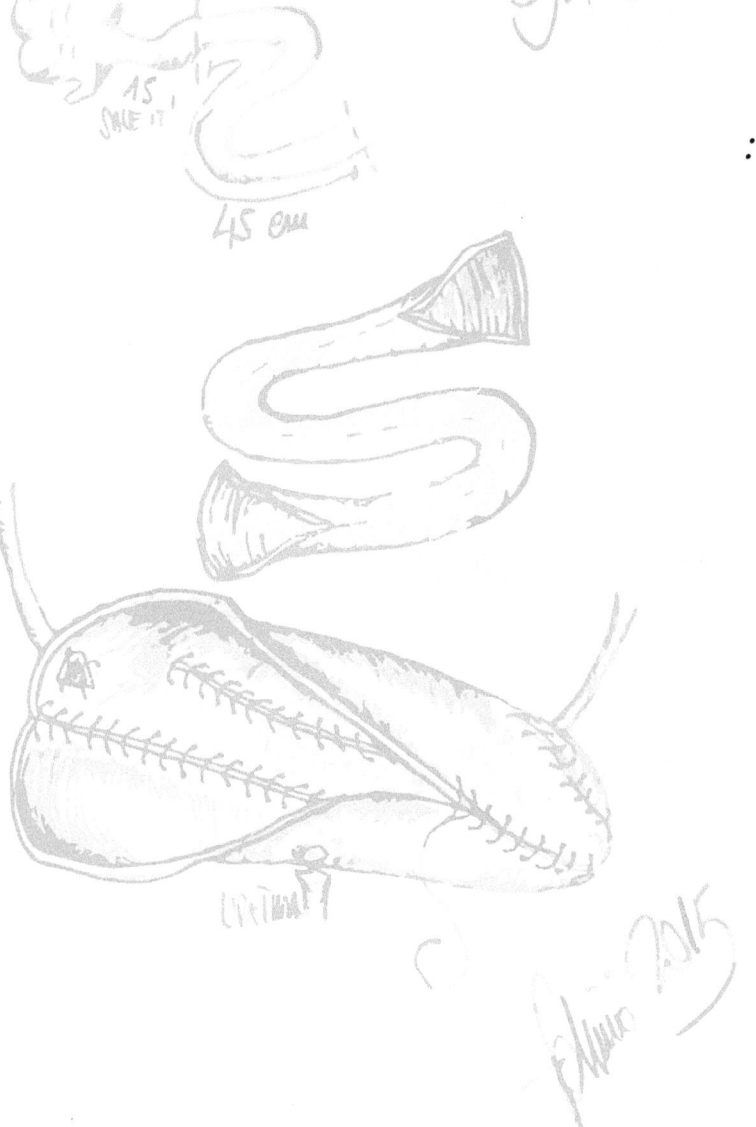

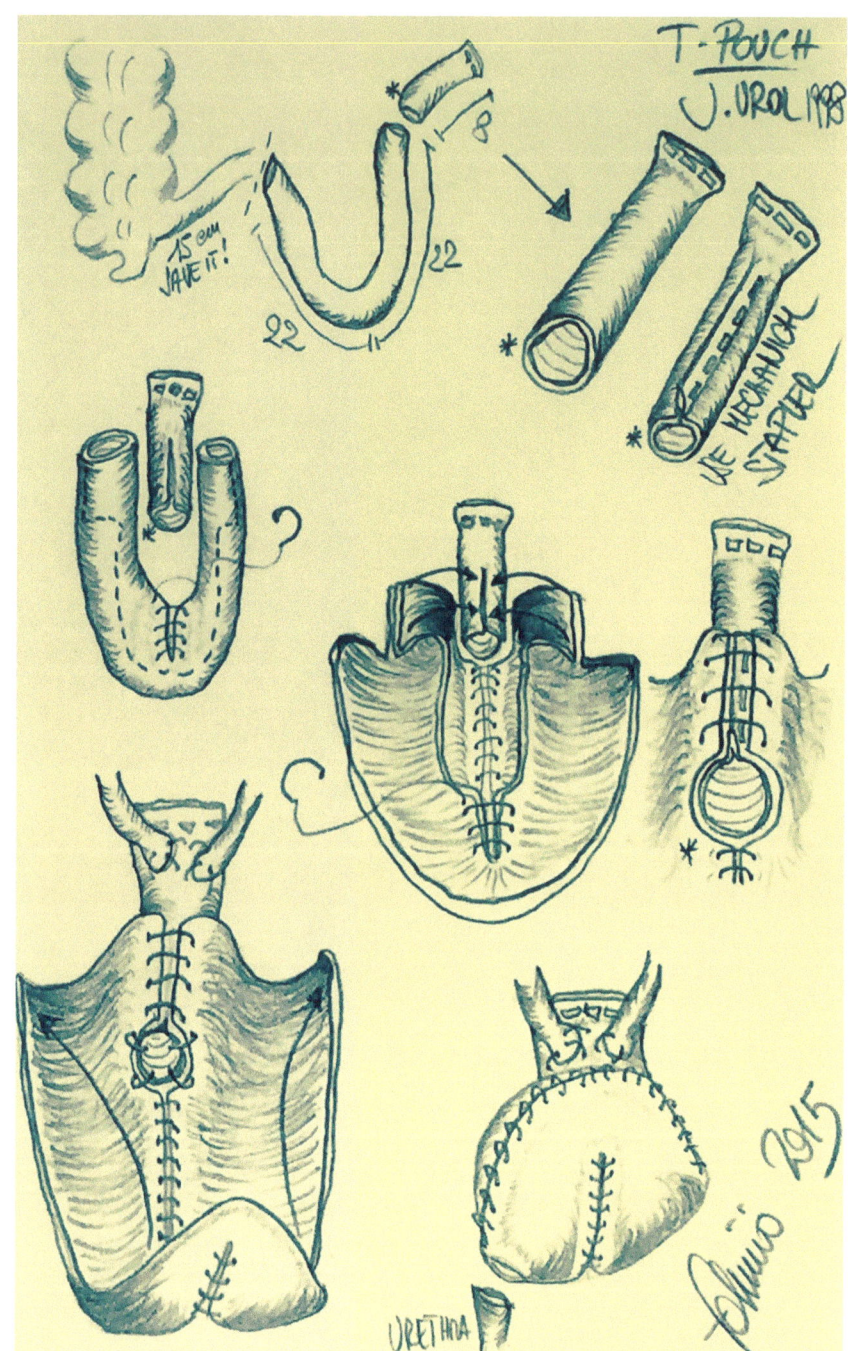

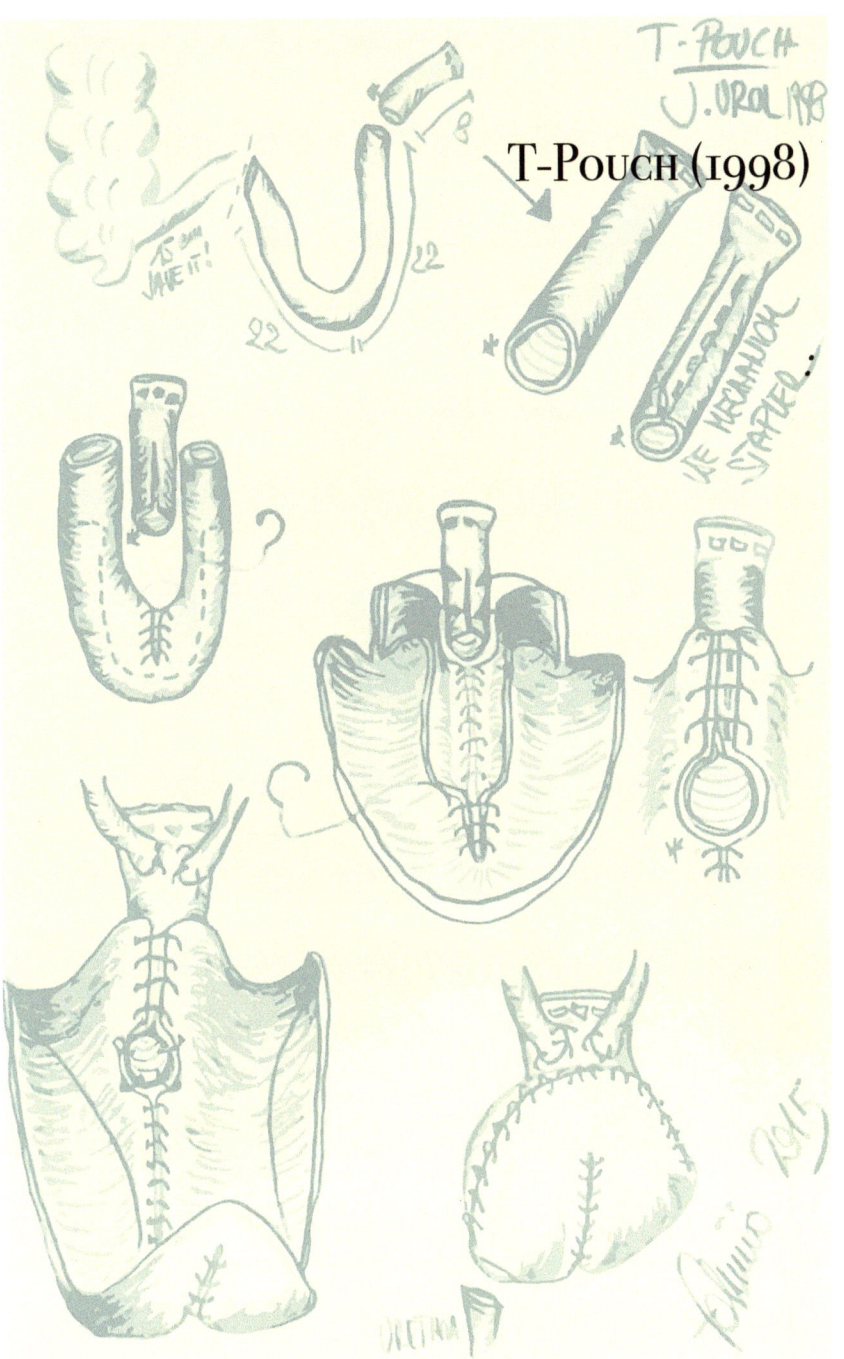

T-Pouch (1998)

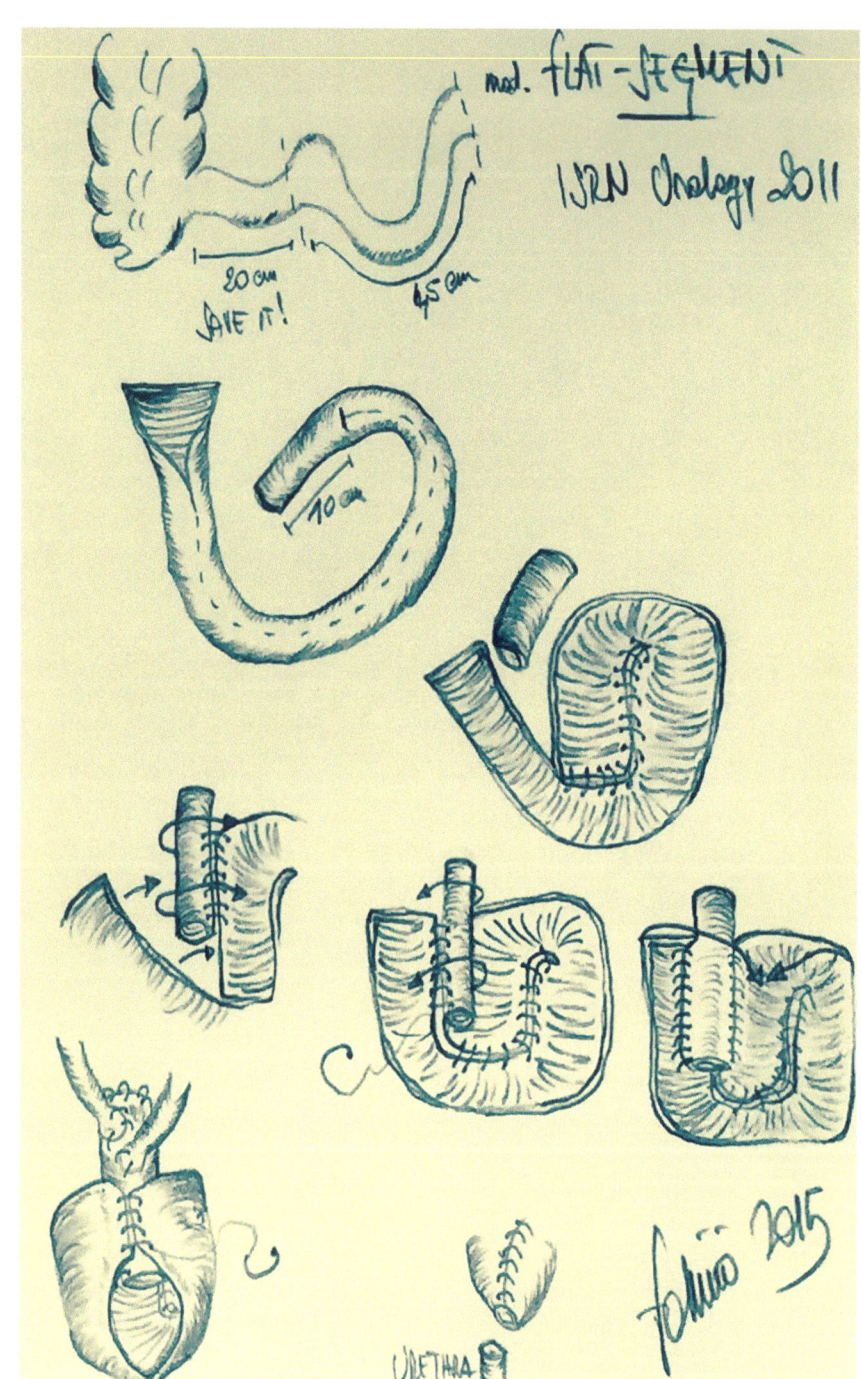

mod. FLAT-SEGMENT

IJRN Urology 2011

20 cm

SAVE IT!

4,5 cm

10 cm

URETHRA

fotino 2015

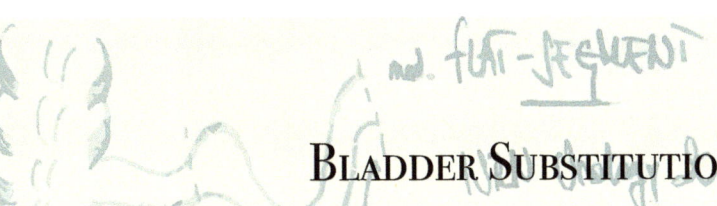

BLADDER SUBSTITUTION
WITH FLAT SEGMENT (MOD. 2011)

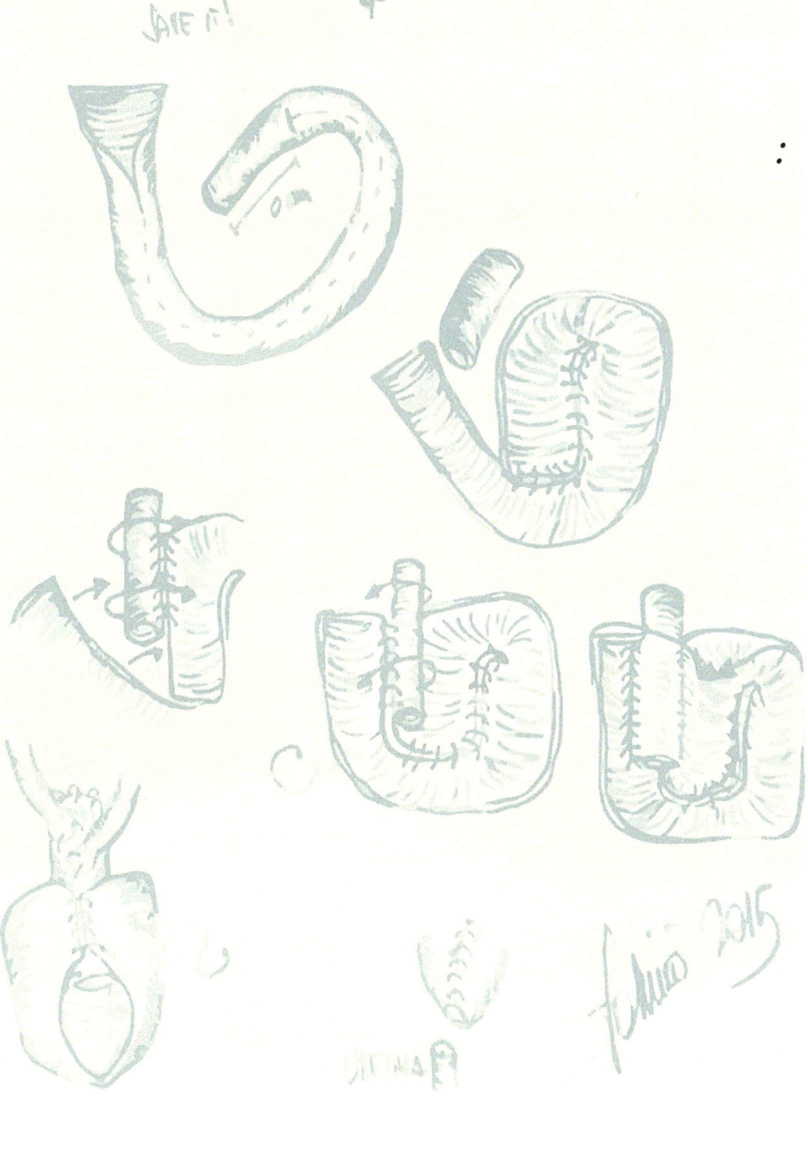

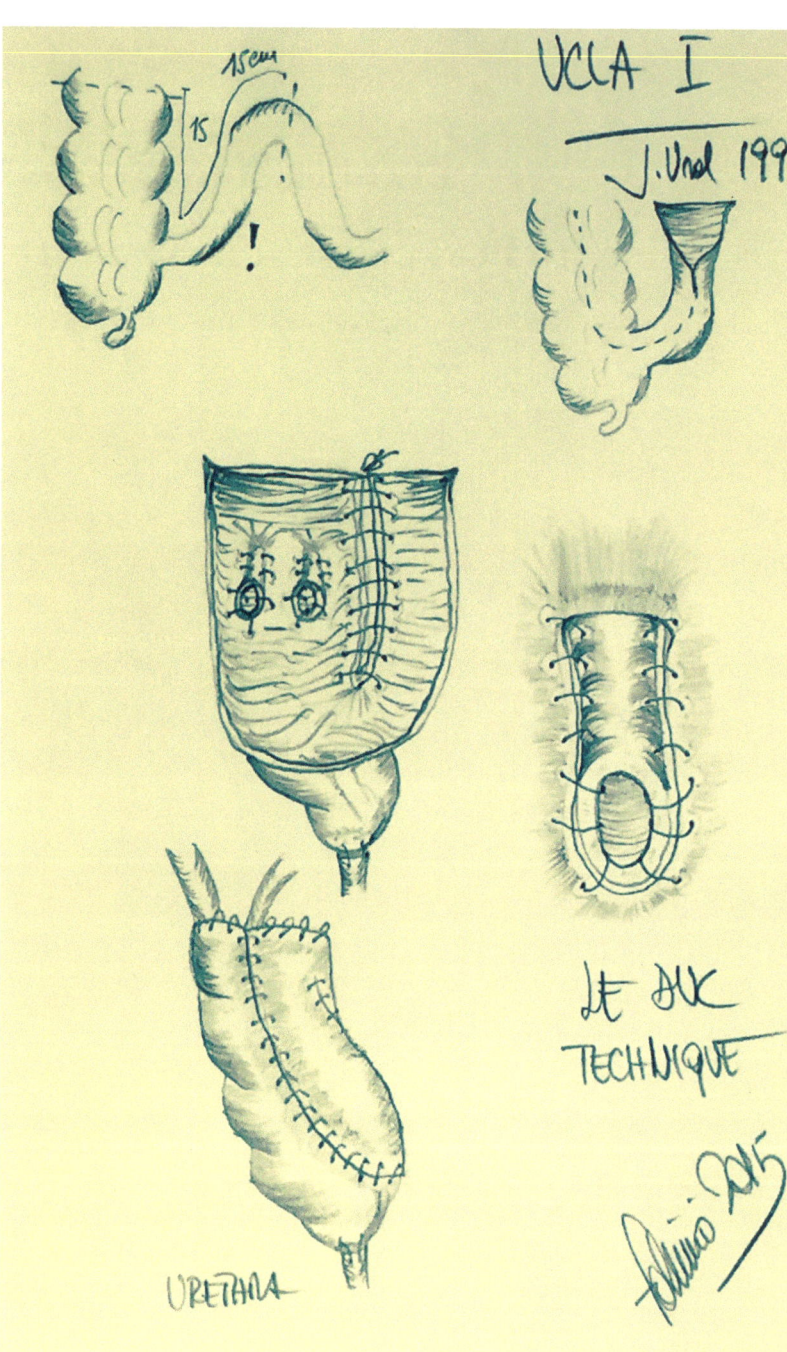

Neobladder UCLA Type I (1994)

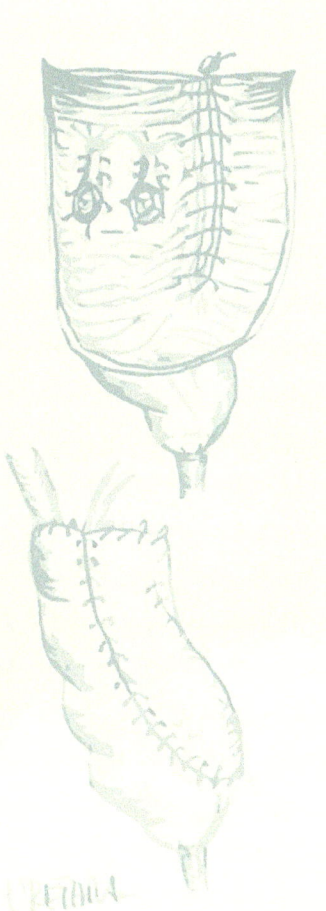

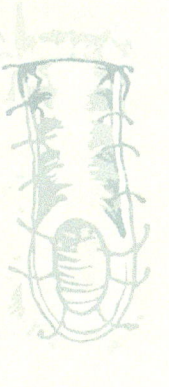

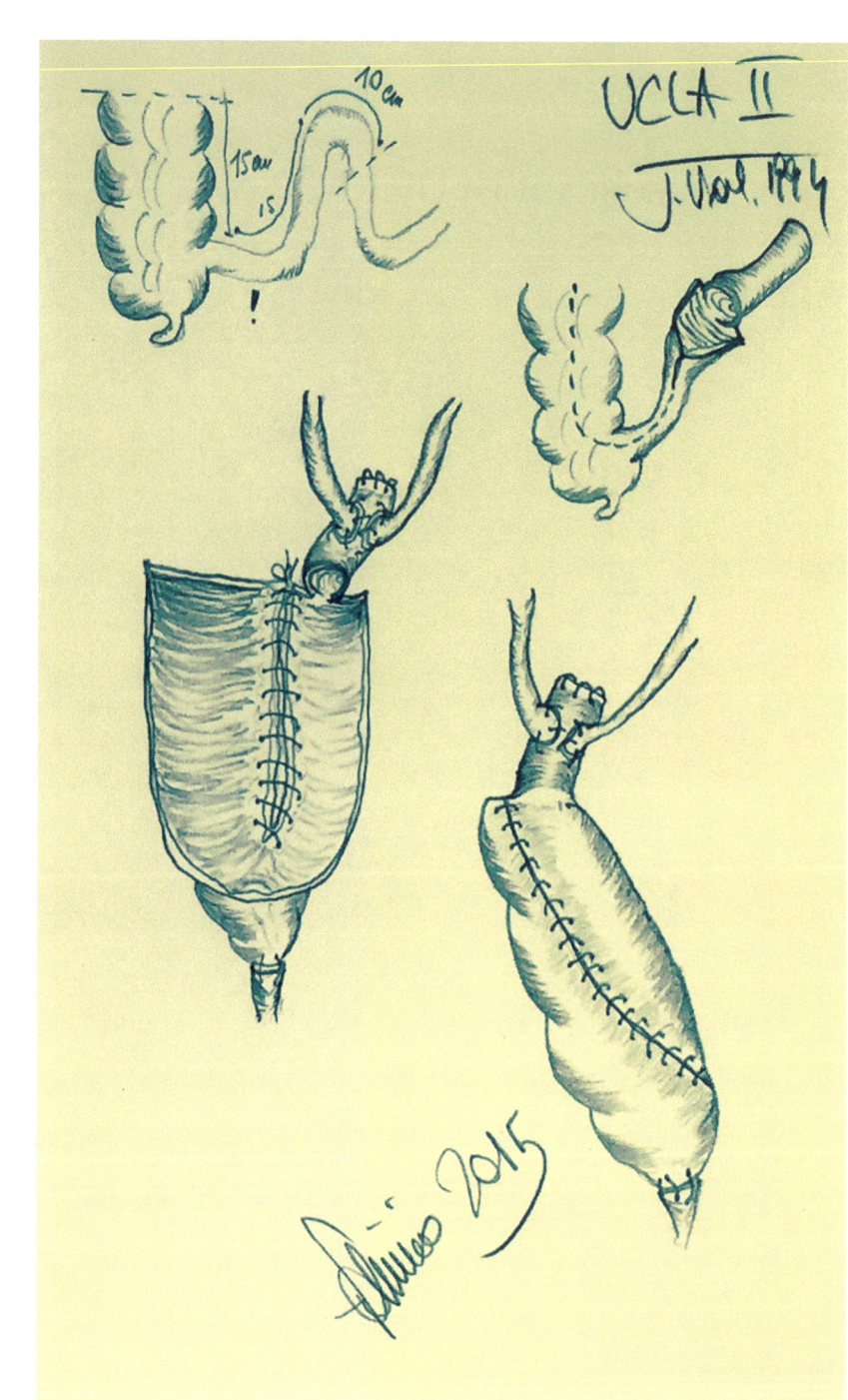

Neobladder UCLA Type II (1994)

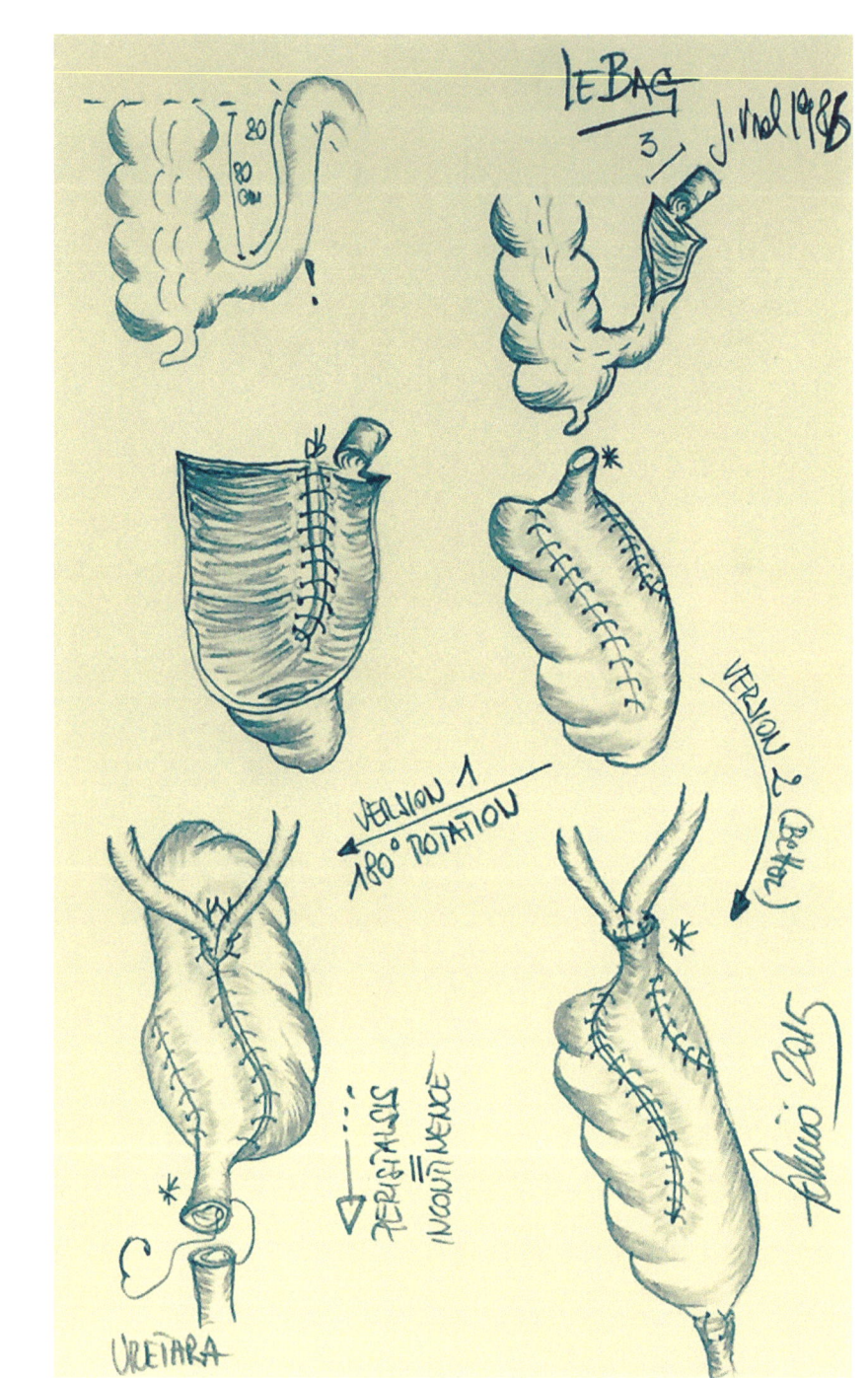

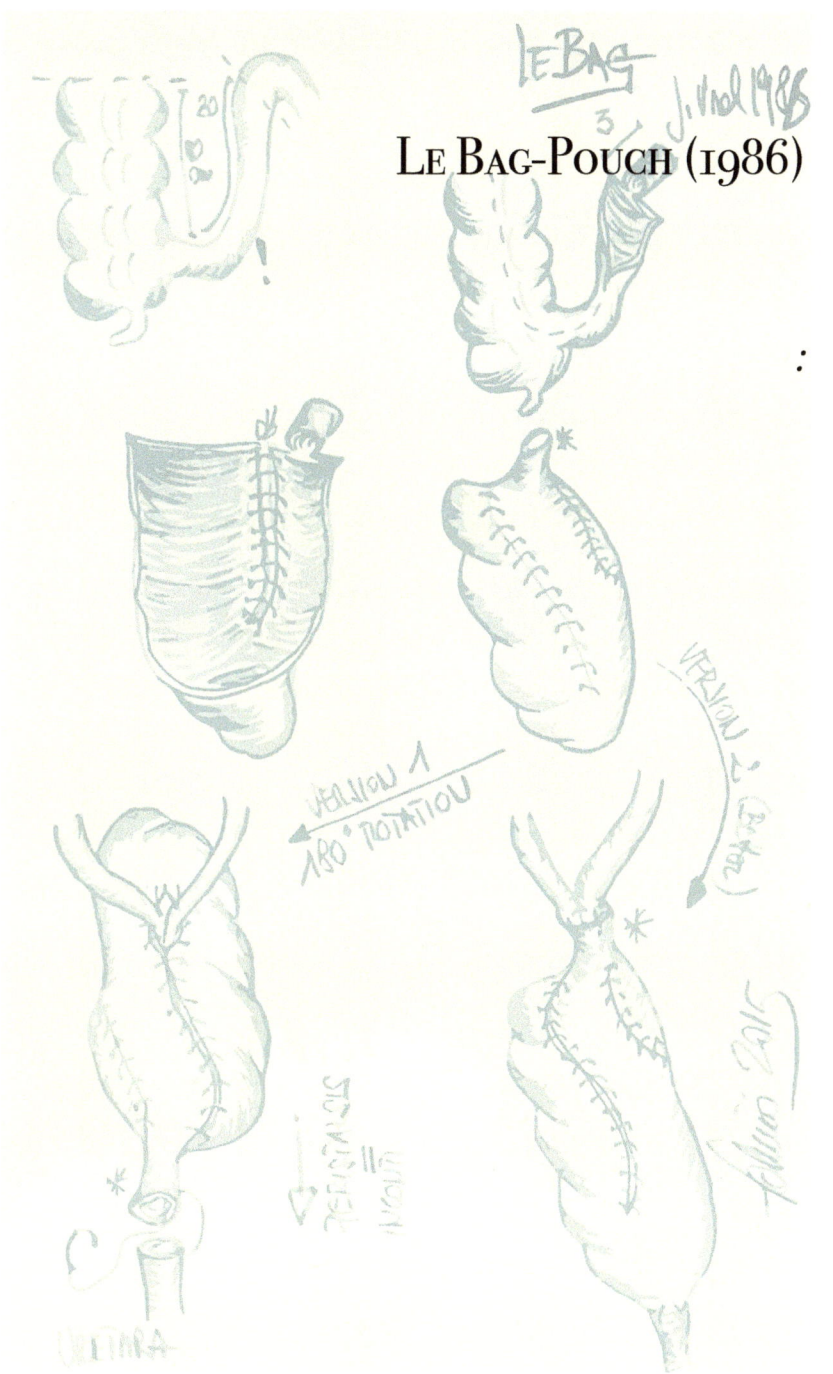

LE BAG-POUCH (1986)

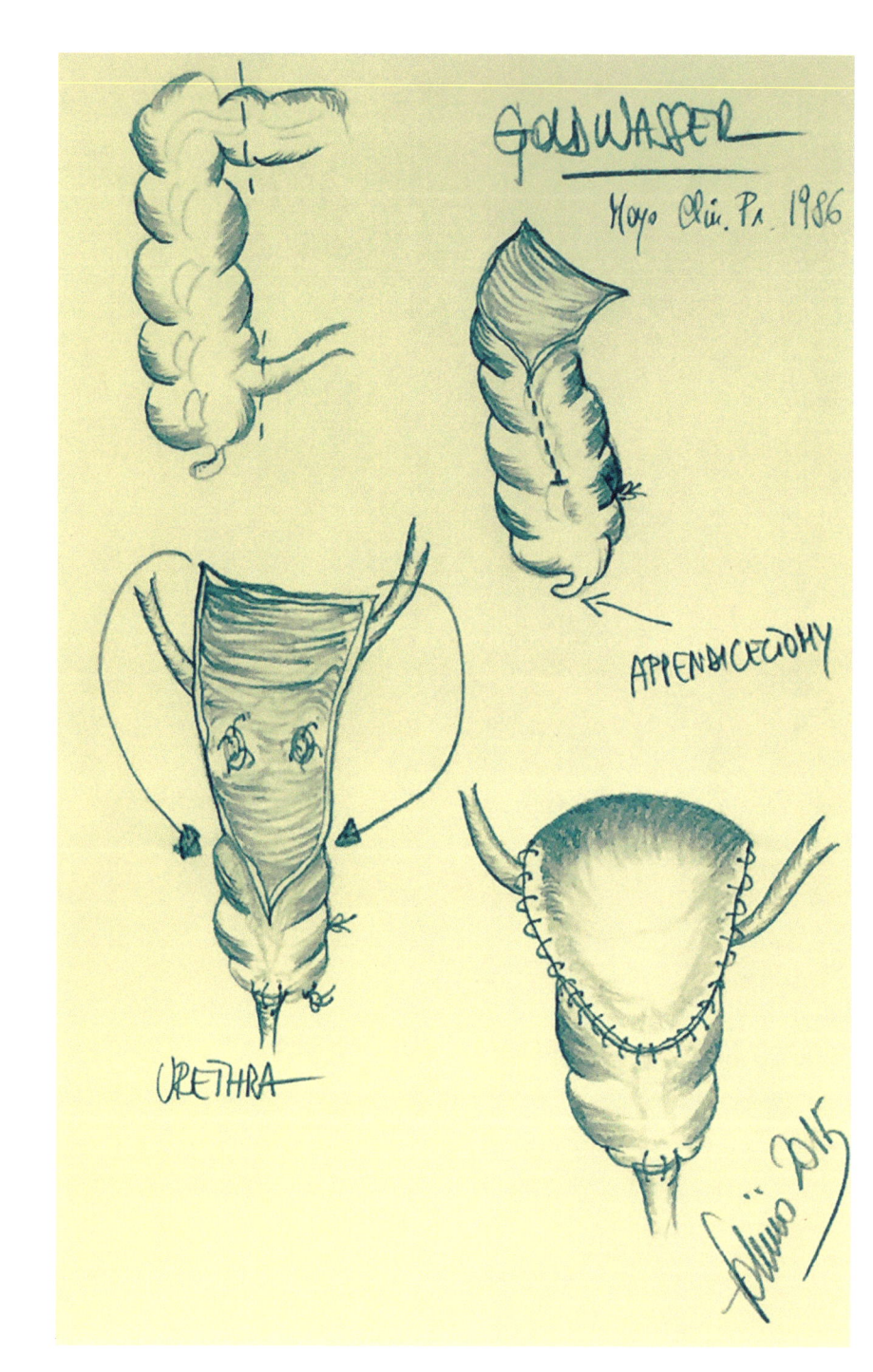

GOLDWASSER

Mayo Clin. Pa. 1986

APPENDICECTOMY

URETHRA

BLADDER SUBSTITUTION
ACCORDING TO GOLDWASSER (1986)

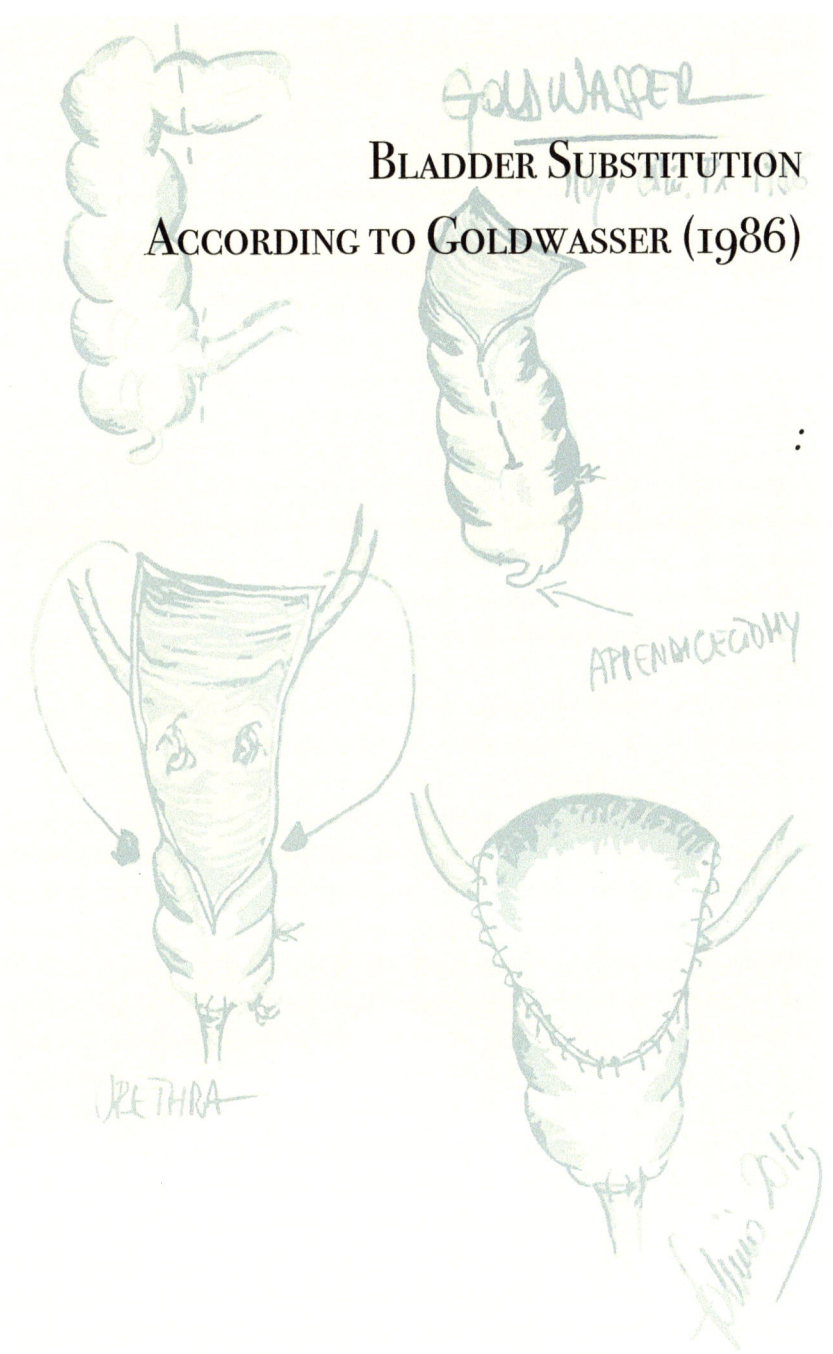

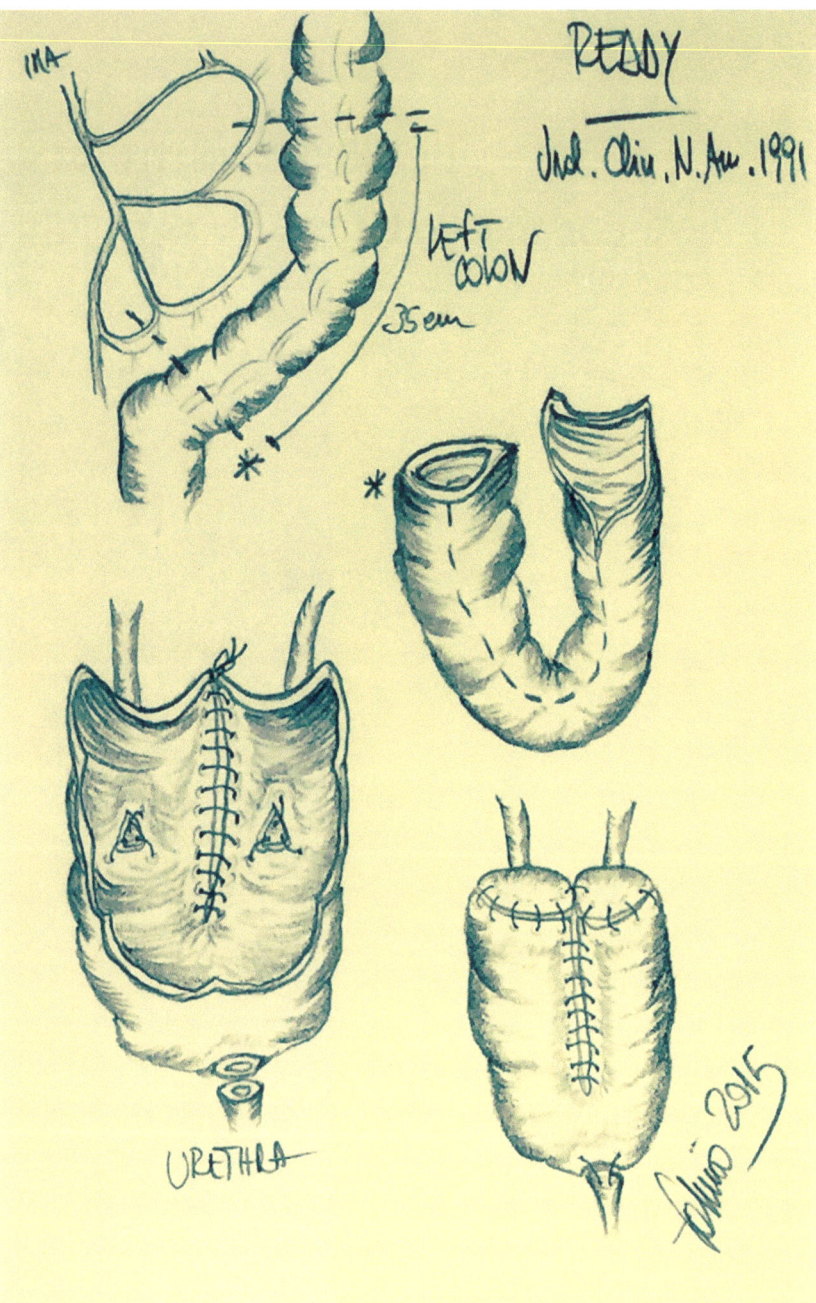

REDDY

Surd. Clin. N. Am. 1991

IMA

LEFT COLON

35 cm

*

*

URETHRA

Shinao 2015

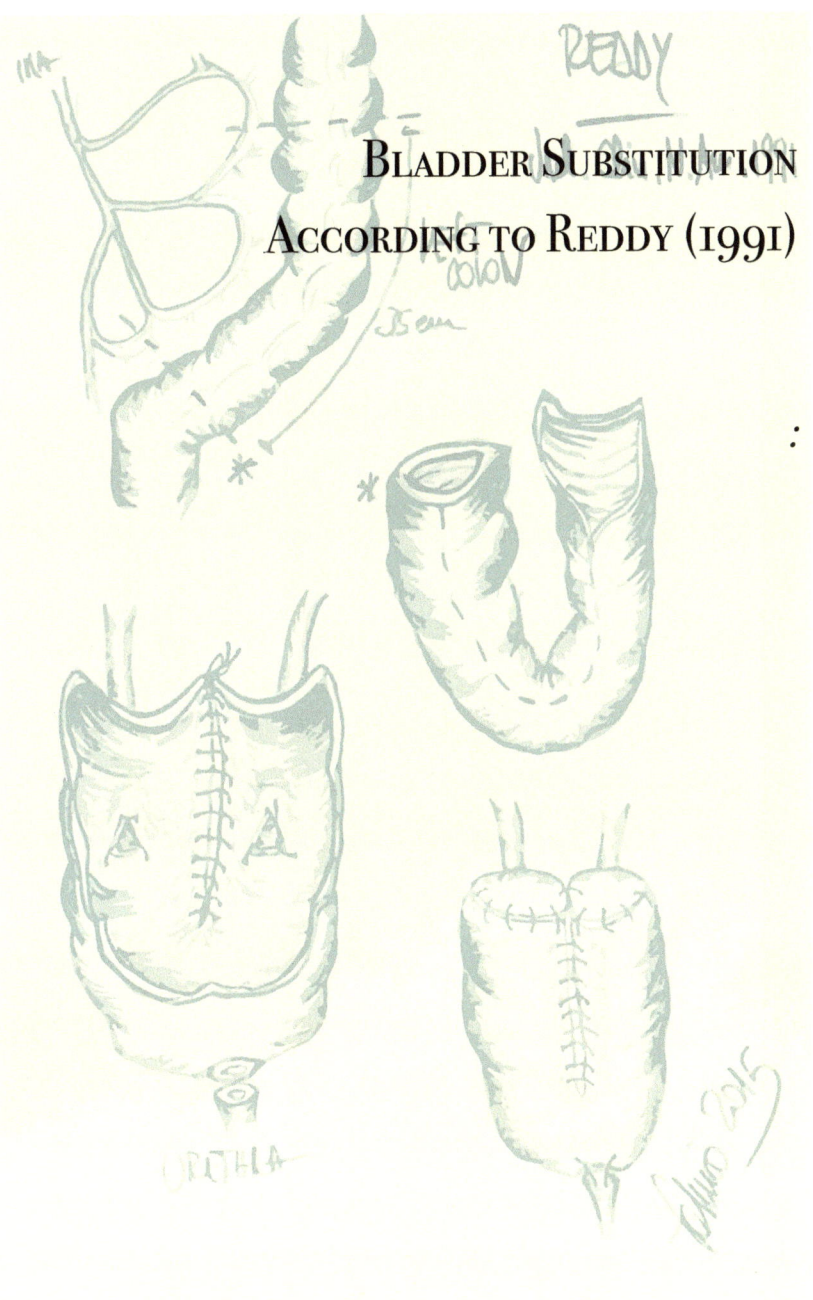

Bladder Substitution According to Reddy (1991)

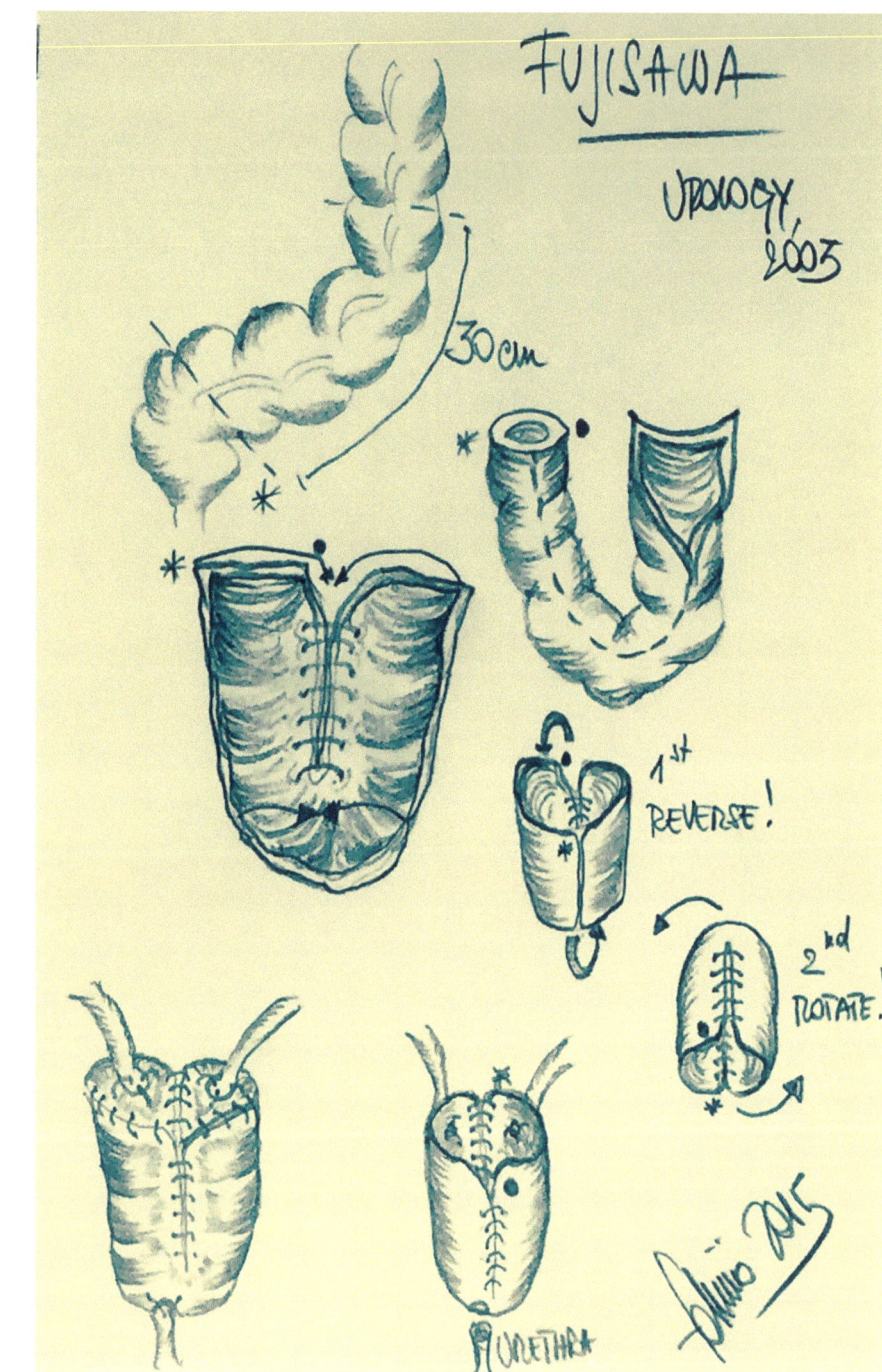

FUJISAWA

UROLOGY,
2003

30 cm

1st REVERSE!

2nd ROTATE!

URETHRA

Bladder Substitution
According to Fujisawa (2003)

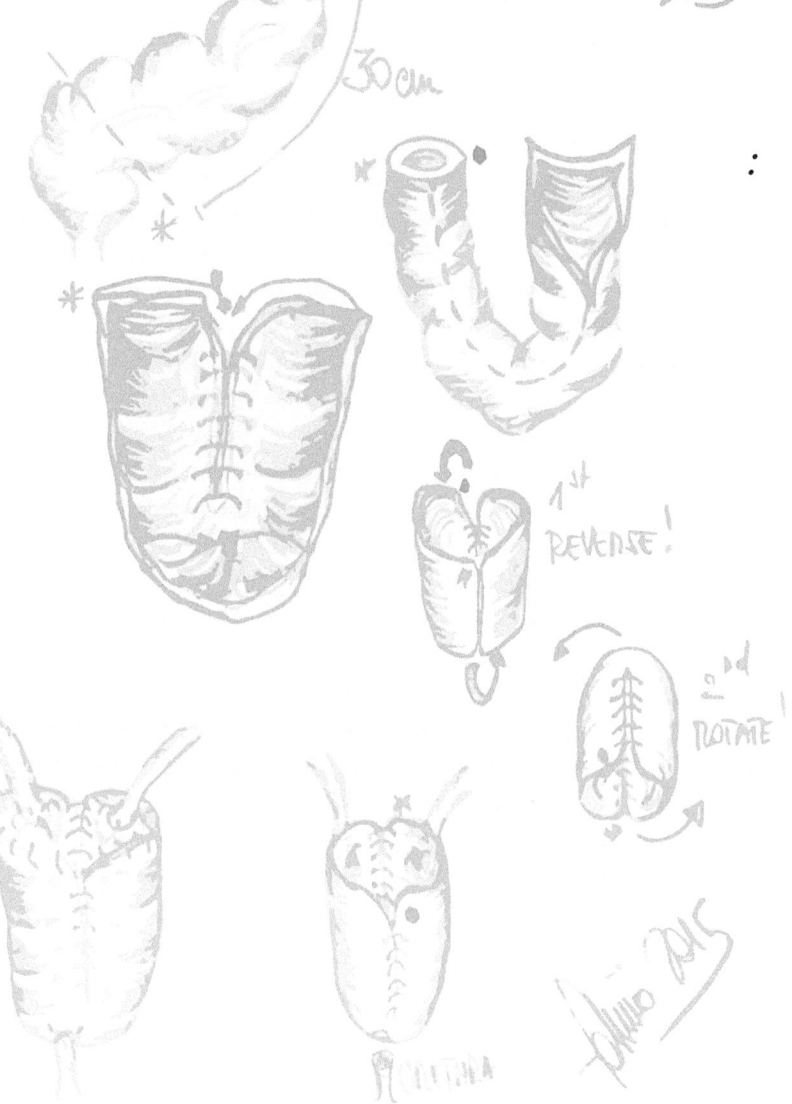

"SPIRAL NEOBLADDER"
Urol. Oncol. 2013

20 cm   15

URETHRA

fabio 2015

Spiral Neobladder (2013)

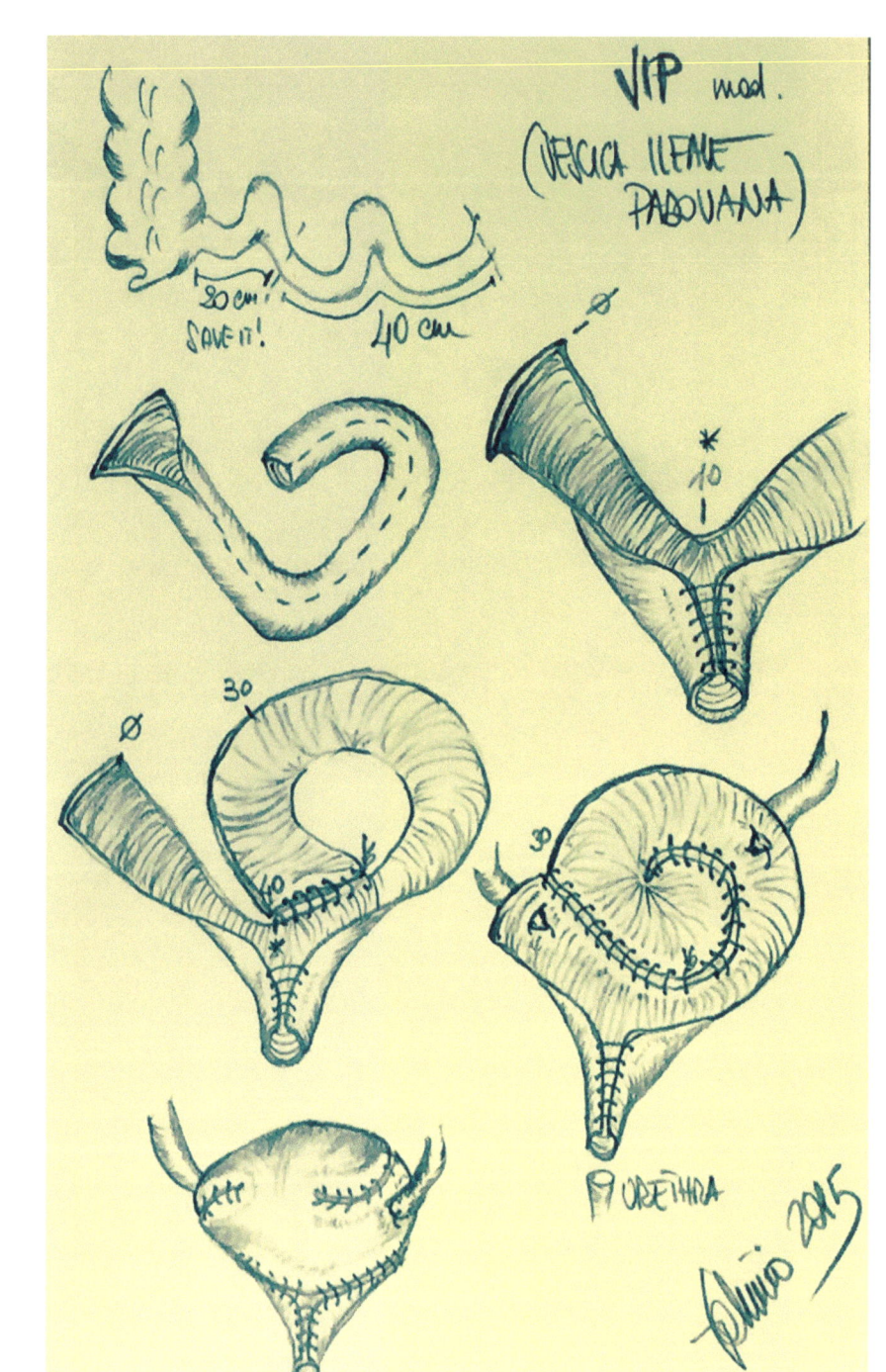

VIP – Vescica Ileale Padovana (1997)

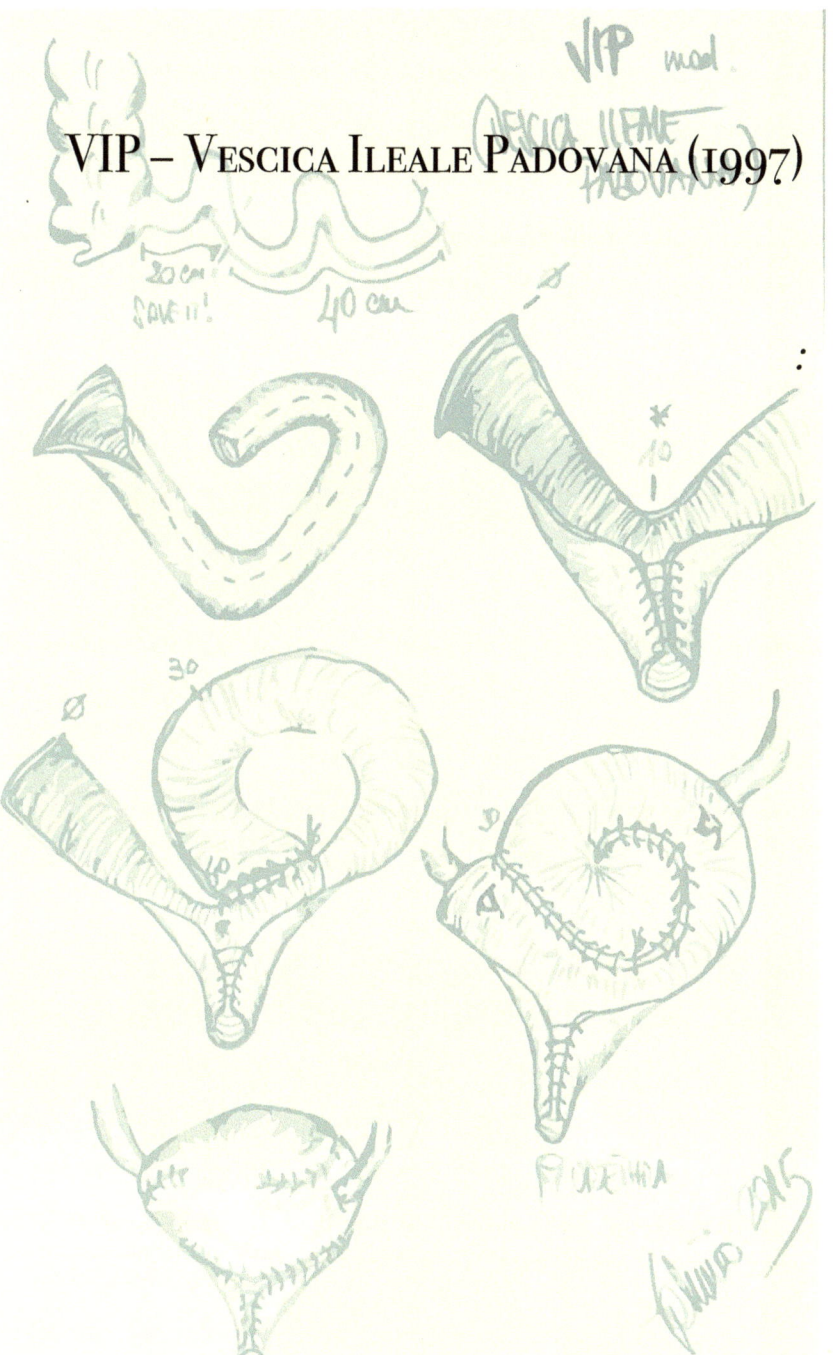

Ves. Pa.

VESICA PATAVINA

ERUS 2015
WCE 2015

20 cm
SAVE IT!

45 cm

40*
40

5 cm

30

-5
0
10

URETHRA

1/2

VES.PA. – VESICA PATAVINA (2015)

... AND IN CASE OF
SHORT LEFT URETER ...

VES. PR. REVENGE

ERUS 2015
WCE 2015

20 cm
SAVE IT

4.5 cm

5 cm

30

FEED

-5
0

URETHRA
10

Olivio 2015

8/2

Ves. Pa. Reverse (2015)

... AND IN ONE OF
SHORT LEFT URETER

VES. PA. REVERSE

FIRUS 2015
WCE 2015

:

20cm
(ARE?)   45cm

5 cm

~5
8

URETHRA
10

30

Silvio 2015

2/2

www.ingramcontent.com/pod-product-compliance
Lightning Source LLC
Chambersburg PA
CBHW040835180526
45159CB00001B/198